SEXUAL EXPLOITATION
IN PROFESSIONAL RELATIONSHIPS

SEXUAL EXPLOITATION
IN PROFESSIONAL RELATIONSHIPS

Edited by

Glen O. Gabbard, M.D.

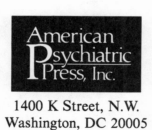

American
Psychiatric
Press, Inc.

1400 K Street, N.W.
Washington, DC 20005

The paper used in this publication meets the minimum requirements of the American National Standard for Information Sciences—Permanence of Paper for Printed Library Materials ANSI Z39.48-1984.   ∞

Library of Congress Cataloging-in-Publication Data

Sexual exploitation in professional relations / edited by Glen O. Gabbard.— 1st ed.
     p.   cm.
Bibliography: p.
Includes index.
ISBN 0-88048-290-7
   1. Psychotherapist and patient. 2. Psychotherapists—Sexual behavior. 3. Sexually abused patients. 4. Psychotherapists—Professional ethics. 5. White collar workers—Sexual behavior.
I. Gabbard, Glen O.
RC480.8.S48 1989
364.1'68—dc19   88-3280
                                                        CIP

Contents

Contributors

Annette M. Brodsky, Ph.D.
Chief Psychologist/Professor
Harbor-UCLA Medical Center
UCLA School of Medicine
Torrance, California

Dean T. Collins, M.D.
Director of Psychiatry
The Menninger Clinic
Topeka, Kansas

Shirley Feldman-Summers, Ph.D.
Licensed psychologist in private practice
Seattle, Washington

Michael Feldstein, Ph.D.
Scientific Director
Frontier Science and Technology
   Research Foundation, Inc.
Brookline, Massachusetts

Glen O. Gabbard, M.D.
Section Chief and Staff Psychoanalyst
The Menninger Clinic
Instructor, Topeka Institute for Psychoanalysis
Faculty, Karl Menninger School of Psychiatry
Topeka, Kansas

Nanette Gartrell, M.D.
Clinical Associate Professor of Psychiatry
UCSF School of Medicine
San Francisco, California

Lucille Gechtman, M.S.W., L.C.S.W.
Licensed Clinical Social Worker
Encino, California

Judith Herman, M.D.
Clinical Assistant Professor of Psychiatry
Harvard Medical School and
   The Cambridge Hospital
Cambridge, Massachusetts

William E. Hulme, Ph.D.
Professor, Pastoral Theology and Ministry
Luther Northwestern Theological Seminary
St. Paul, Minnesota

Russell Localio, J.D., M.P.H., M.S.
Project Director, Medical Practice Study
Harvard University
Cambridge, Massachusetts

Carol C. Nadelson, M.D.
Professor and Vice Chairman
Department of Psychiatry
New England Medical Center Hospitals
Boston, Massachusetts
Editor-in-Chief
American Psychiatric Press, Inc.
Washington, D.C.

Silvia Olarte, M.D.
Clinical Associate Professor of Psychiatry
New York Medical College
New York, New York

Irwin N. Perr, M.D., J.D.
Professor of Psychiatry
Robert Wood Johnson Medical School
University of Medicine and Dentistry of New Jersey
Piscataway, New Jersey

Kenneth S. Pope, Ph.D.
Independent practice
Los Angeles, California

Leslie Schover, Ph.D.
Head, Section of Psychosexual Disorders
Departments of Psychiatry and Urology
The Cleveland Clinic Foundation
Cleveland, Ohio

Sydney Smith, Ph.D.
Senior Staff Psychologist
Division of Law and Psychiatry
The Menninger Foundation
Topeka, Kansas

Janet L. Sonne, M.D.
Staff Psychologist and Instructor
Department of Psychiatry
Loma Linda University Medical Center
Loma Linda, California

Stuart W. Twemlow, M.D.
Private practice of psychiatry
Topeka, Kansas

Acknowledgments

The authors gratefully acknowledge permission to reprint portions of the following material:

Chapter 1

Gartrell N, Herman J, Olarte S, et al: Psychiatrist-patient sexual contact: results of a national survey, I: prevalence. Am J Psychiatry 143:1126–1131, 1986.

Chapter 9

Gabbard GO, Pope KS: Sexual intimacies after termination: clinical, ethical, and legal aspects. The Independent Practitioner 8:21–26, 1988.

Introduction

The problem of incest has lurched into public awareness over the last decade or so. Clinicians have noted a prevalence rate as high as 30–33 percent (Rosenfeld 1979; Spencer 1978) in outpatient caseloads. The devastating effects of incest have also been more fully appreciated (Gelinas 1983). In parallel with this increased interest has been a growing awareness of another form of incest—sexual exploitation of patients, clients, students, and others by professionals. The victims of this form of professional incest have placed their trust in a person whom they assume will place their interests above his or her own by the very nature of the professional relationship. When this trust is betrayed, the impact is often as damaging as familial incest.

The analogy to incest is appropriate for a number of reasons. Incest victims and those who have been sexually exploited by professionals have remarkably similar symptoms: shame, intense guilt associated with a feeling that they were somehow responsible for their victimization, feelings of isolation and forced silence, poor self-esteem, suicidal and/or self-destructive behavior, and denial. Reactions of friends and family—disbelief, discounting, embarrassment—are also similar in both groups. Most fundamentally, professional relationships are characterized by the development of a powerful transference element in which a parent-child relationship is unconsciously reestablished. Hence, sexual relationships under such circumstances are always symbolically incestuous (Barnhouse 1978).

Sexual boundary violations involving psychotherapists and patients have become a major concern to the professions of psychiatry and psychology. Surveys (Gartrell et al. 1986; Holroyd and Brodsky 1977; Pope et al. 1979, 1986, 1987) have documented a prevalence rate as high as 10–12 percent among male therapists. Concern has been expressed about the possibility of an underlying sexism in psychotherapy training and practice (Karasu 1980) that may be reflected in the fact that the overwhelming majority of offending therapists are male. Legal sanctions and ethics committee actions have been advocated by the professions of psychiatry, psychology, and social work (Pope 1986a, 1986b; Stone 1976). About one-third of the states have made therapist-patient sexual relations illegal.

A survey of practitioners (Bouhoutsos et al. 1983) has demonstrated that at least 90 percent of patients are seriously harmed by this form of sexual exploitation. Beyond the harm done to patients, the reputation of the psychotherapeutic professions is tarnished each time the media publicizes a criminal proceeding based on sexual boundary violations (Webb 1986). The problem of sexual exploitation is one with which every clinician must be familiar. It is estimated that over one-half of all therapists will treat patients who have been sexually involved with prior treaters (Pope and Bouhoutsos 1986). If one expands the estimate to include sexual exploitation involving nonpsychotherapeutic professional relationships, the figure would have to be revised considerably upwards.

While a good deal of attention has been devoted to therapist-patient sex, sexual exploitation in other professional relationships still remains under a shroud of secrecy to a large extent. Unlike the mental health professionals, attorneys and chiropractors, for example, do not even have ethical codes prohibiting sexual involvement with clients and patients. There is little in the literature about forms of sexual exploitation that lie outside the psychotherapeutic realm. This volume is an attempt to bring more attention to all varieties of professional sexual exploitation in recognition of the fact that transference is not confined to the psychotherapeutic setting (Brenner 1982). Transference is pervasive in professional relationships. Even beyond transference considerations, there are other compelling reasons that sexual exploitation is damaging within such a context. The contributors to this volume have considered those reasons in some detail.

Section One is devoted to therapist-patient sexual exploitation. It is more extensive than Section Two simply because much more is known about this form of sexual exploitation than about others. The first three chapters consider the prevalence of the problem in each of the three major professions that practice psychotherapy. In Chapter 1, Gartrell et al. report their findings from a national survey of U.S. psychiatrists. Brodsky summarizes the data from the four large-scale studies of psychologists in Chapter 2. In Chapter 3, Gechtman's national survey of social workers—the only one of its kind—appears in print for the first time. The strikingly lower incidence of sexual exploitation in the social work profession raises some provocative questions. Although self-report questionnaire studies are fraught with methodological problems, these surveys are more likely to underestimate the scope of the problem than to exaggerate it. At the very least, they suggest that the mental health professions have a significant problem on their hands. Chapter 4 documents in detail the devastating consequences of therapist-patient sex. Pope suggests that there are at least 10 common characteristics of victims, which taken together constitute a "therapist-patient sex syndrome." Here again the similarities with incest (and with posttraumatic stress disorder) are clear.

Chapters 5 and 6 are psychoanalytic perspectives on the dynamics of therapist-patient sex. In Chapter 5, Smith describes two frequent childhood scenarios of the female patient who is likely to be exploited by her therapist. Via the repetition compulsion and the regression inherent in transference, these past scenarios are reenacted in the present. The therapist who colludes with this reenactment identifies with the sadistic father from the patient's past rather than interpreting the patient's tendency to repeat in action what ought to be only verbalized and understood. In Chapter 6, Twemlow and Gabbard examine the phenomenon of lovesickness in the psychotherapist. How is it that otherwise respectable professionals sacrifice their careers and marriages for the "true love" they feel for a patient?

Treatment of victims of therapist-patient sex is discussed in Chapters 7 and 8. Pope and Gabbard outline principles of individual psychotherapy to help subsequent therapists work with patients who have been betrayed once and find it difficult to trust again. In Chapter 8, Sonne shares her experience working as a group therapist with the UCLA Post-Therapy Support Groups designed specifically for victims of sexual abuse by therapists. Gabbard and Pope collaborate again in Chapter 9 on an area of major controversy: Is sex after termination of therapy ever acceptable or ethical? The authors present seven reasons why there can only be one answer: Once a patient, always a patient. Finally, in Chapter 10, Pope provides some guidelines on treating exploitative therapists.

In Section Two, we consider forms of sexual exploitation outside traditional psychotherapy. Sexual contact with sex therapists, ironically, is rarely reported. In Chapter 11, Schover presents reasons why this problem may be less of an occupational hazard for sex therapists than for others. She also discusses the decline of sex surrogates in the field.

Another area that has received scant attention in the literature is sexual relations between psychiatric hospital staff and the inpatients they treat. In Chapter 12, Collins draws a profile of the susceptible patient and another of the staff member likely to be exploitative, based on his extensive review of sexual boundary violations in a variety of hospital settings. Chapter 13, also contributed by Pope, looks at sexual intimacy between teachers and students. In Chapter 14, Hulme writes about sexual boundary crossing in the clergy and the unique aspects of that form of sexual exploitation.

A *fiduciary relationship* is defined as a situation in which one person accepts the trust and confidence of another to act in the latter's best interest. Feldman-Summers, in Chapter 15, uses this concept to examine the similarities of several forms of sexual exploitation. In her series of cases, whether the exploiter was an attorney, a chiropractor, a gynecologist, a mental health counselor, a psychiatrist, or a high school teacher, the negative impact on the victim was strikingly similar, lending further support to her 1984 study (with Jones) on the deleterious effects of exploitation by health care professionals. In Chapter 16, Perr provides an overview of the legal consequences of sexual exploitation. Regardless of the presence or absence of ethical codes, all professionals—including dentists, attorneys, judges, and others—have been censured by civil proceedings, ethics committees, and licensing boards. He informs the reader of a growing trend, already completed in several states, to criminalize penalties for therapist-patient sex. Finally, Nadelson provides some thoughtful comments about the significance of the phenomena described in this book.

The contributors to this volume all owe a debt of gratitude to the victims of sexual exploitation who have courageously come forth and have spoken up about the unspeakable. I personally wish to make several acknowledgments: to the Menninger Clinic, for providing moral and financial support; to Alice Brand, chief librarian of the Menninger Library, for her assistance in providing me up-to-date literature reviews; to Mary Ann Clifft for her meticulous proofreading and her careful preparation of the index; to Dr. Ken Pope for his numerous helpful suggestions at all stages of this project; and to Faye Schoenfeld, my extraordinarily patient secretary, who typed numerous drafts of the chapters and worked her way through a complicated web of software deriving from an equally complicated web of mismatched word processors.

Glen O. Gabbard, M.D.

SECTION ONE

Chapter 1

Prevalence of Psychiatrist-Patient Sexual Contact

Nanette Gartrell, M.D.
Judith Herman, M.D.
Silvia Olarte, M.D.
Michael Feldstein, Ph.D.
Russell Localio, J.D., M.P.H., M.S.

Sexual contact between psychiatrist and patient is explicitly prohibited by the Hippocratic oath and the American Psychiatric Association code of ethics (American Psychiatric Association 1985; Edelstein 1943). Nevertheless, some psychiatrists do become sexually involved with their patients. Professional liability insurance carriers have noted a sharp increase in the number of malpractice claims for sexual misconduct filed in recent years against psychiatrists (APA malpractice claim 1983). Likewise, sexual misconduct complaints to American Psychiatric Association ethics committees have multiplied in the past decade (Moore 1985). Despite the increase in malpractice claims and ethics committee complaints, the prevalence of psychiatrist-patient sexual contact has never been reliably documented; existing estimates are based on a few small or geographically restricted surveys. Kardener and associates (1973), for example, found in a random sample of male physicians in Los Angeles that 10 percent of 114 psychiatrists engaged in sexual contact with their patients. In replications of the Kardener study that surveyed female physicians, Perry (1976) reported that no female psychiatrist among 30 respondents had engaged in sexual contact with patients.

There have been several surveys of psychologists regarding therapist-patient sexual contact, all of which are discussed in Chapter 2. Bouhoutsos et al. (1983) surveyed all licensed psychologists in California. Of the 704 respondents (16 percent return rate), significantly more men (4.8 percent) than women (0.8 percent) had been sexually involved with patients. The 704 respondents had treated a total of 559 patients who had been sexually involved with previous therapists. When asked to assess the effects of the prior involvement on their patients, the respondents indicated that 90 percent of the patients suffered ill effects. Eleven percent of these patients were hospitalized as a result of the sexual involvement, and 1 percent committed suicide.

We undertook this study to obtain data on psychiatrist-patient sexual contact by means of a large-scale national survey. The survey was designed to assess psychiatrists' attitudes about sexual contact with patients and to determine the prevalence of sexual misconduct among respondents. We hypothesized that there would be differences between male and female psychiatrists with respect to sexual misconduct. We also speculated that offenders would be divided into two groups: one-time violators who are remorseful about their sexual involvement with a patient and repeat offenders for whom the sexual misconduct is ego syntonic and highly rationalized. In this chapter, we present data on the respondents' demographic characteristics, their sexual contacts with their own patients, and their sexual contacts with their own therapists.

METHOD

A 34-item questionnaire contained 9 items on the demographic characteristics of the respondents, 4 items on attitudes toward psychiatrist-patient sexual contact, and 21 items on respondents' personal experiences with their own patients. Sexual contact was defined as "contact which was intended to arouse or satisfy sexual desire in the patient, therapist, or both." Respondents were asked to restrict their answers to adult patients; an adult was defined as "a person who has reached the legal age of consent for sexual relations" in the respondent's state of residence. Included in the questions on personal experience were 2 items requesting information on patients who had been sexually involved with their previous therapists and who were subsequently treated by the respondents and 1 item inquiring whether the respondents had had sexual relationships with their own therapists. The remainder of the personal experience questions focused on the respondents' sexual contacts with their own patients. Respondents were asked to specify the number of male and female patients with whom they had been sexually involved. Those who answered affirmatively to sexual involvement with patients were then asked a series of questions about their most recent sexual contact. Most of the questions required a precoded, forced-choice response (yes/no or always appropriate/sometimes appropriate/always inappropriate) or a numerical specification. Space was provided for additional comments. The questionnaire was extensively reviewed by numerous psychiatrists, biostatisticians, and survey experts before it was distributed.

The questionnaire, a one-page cover letter, and a stamped, addressed return envelope were mailed out in November 1984 to 5,574 psychiatrists. The sample was selected by taking every fifth name from the 27,875 psychiatrists in the United States who were under the age of 65 years listed alphabetically in the American Medical Association (AMA) Masterfile. The cover letter explained the purpose of the study, the nature of the selection process, and the procedures for establishing confidentiality. The anonymous responses were keypunched and tabulated. Unless otherwise noted in the text, we used χ^2 tests (without continuity correction) in the analysis; we used Fisher's exact test (two-tailed) in all cases for which expected cell frequencies were too small for accurate use of χ^2 as a test of significance (Armitage 1971).

RESULTS

Characteristics of the Respondents

Questionnaires were returned by 1,442 (26 percent) of the psychiatrists before the June 1985 deadline. The returns included 19 uncompleted questionnaires with obscenities or other hostile comments written on them (12 objecting to the fact that the cover letter and questionnaire did not condemn psychiatrist-patient sexual contact and seven objecting to being surveyed about a topic that these respondents considered unimportant), which were eliminated from the data base. In addition, 30 questionnaires were returned by the postal service because of incorrect addresses. The results we report are based on replies from 1,423 respondents: 291 female (20 percent) and 1,124 male (79 percent) psychiatrists and 8 whose sex was unspecified. The total number of responses for each question varied because some respondents did not answer all questions.

We compared the respondents' age, gender, and board certification status with those of the psychiatrists in the 1983 AMA Masterfile (Table 1). The respondents were nearly identical in gender and age distribution to the population of the Masterfile, although they included slightly more younger and slightly fewer older psychiatrists. A significantly greater proportion of the respondents than of the whole population of psychiatrists were board certified.

Seventy-six percent of the respondents were married, and an additional 4.6 percent were involved in committed relationships. Eleven percent were single, 7.8 percent were separated or divorced, and 0.9 percent were widowed. Ninety-five percent of the respondents specified their sexual orientation as heterosexual, 2.8 percent homosexual, and 2 percent bisexual. Eighty-four percent of the respondents were American Psychiatric Association members.

Sixty-seven percent of the respondents had been in psychotherapy or psychoanalysis. Of these 942 respondents, 16 percent had been in treatment less than 1 year, 41 percent from 1 to 4 years, and 43 percent for more than 4 years. Eighty-seven percent of the respon-

Table 1. Characteristics of Respondents to a Questionnaire on Sexual Contact with Patients and of Psychiatrists in the 1983 AMA Masterfile

Characteristics	Psychiatrists in AMA Masterfile		Respondents[a]		χ^2	Significance
	n	%	n	%		
Sex						
Female	5,832	19	291	20	2.5[b]	NS
Male	24,931	81	1,124	79		
Age (years)[c]						
Under 35	6,128	22	349	25	13.6[d]	p<.005
35–44	8,725	31	460	32		
45–54	7,343	26	353	25		
55–64	5,849	21	252	18		
Board certification						
Certified	14,941	49	806	57	43.3[b]	p<.001
Not certified	15,822	51	605	43		

[a] Total number of respondents for each characteristic differs because not all respondents answered all questions.
[b] df=1.
[c] Mean ± SD age of respondents, 43.2 ± 10.2 years.
[d] df=3.

dents reported that they had completed an accredited residency. The respondents' years in practice were as follows: 0–5 years, 33 percent; 6–10 years, 20.4 percent; 11–15 years, 16.5 percent; 16–20 years, 12 percent; 21 or more years, 18 percent; the mean ± SD was 11.2 ± 9.0 years.

Sexual Contact with Patients

Eighty-four (6.4 percent) of the 1,316 respondents who answered the question acknowledged having had sexual contact with their own patients. Nine of the respondents were psychiatric residents at the time of sexual contact. We compared the offenders with the nonoffenders on all demographic variables and found that the offenders were more likely to be male ($\chi^2 = 5.5$, df = 1, p < .02), to have completed an accredited residency ($\chi^2 = 5.4$, df = 1, p < .025), and to have undergone personal psychotherapy or psychoanalysis ($\chi^2 = 11.7$, df = 1, p < .001).

The 75 male (7.1 percent, n = 1,057) and 8 female (3.1 percent, n = 257) offenders and 1 whose sex was unspecified acknowledged sexual involvement with a total of 144 patients. Fifty-six of the offenders (66.7 percent) had been involved with 1 patient, and 28 (33.3 percent) with more than 1—17 with 2 patients and 11 with 3 or more patients. The largest number of patients reported involved with 1 offender was 12. All offenders who admitted contact with more than 1 patient were male; the gender difference in repeat offenses was statistically significant (Fisher's exact test, p < .05, two-tailed). Eighty-eight percent of the contacts for which both the psychiatrist's and the patient's gender were specified occurred between male psychiatrists and female patients, 3.5 percent between female psychiatrists and male patients, and 1.4 percent between female psychiatrists and female patients.

The 84 offenders provided detailed information about their most recent experience of sexual contact with a patient. The patients (n = 84) ranged in age from 20 to 48 years, with a mean ± SD of 33 ± 6.9 years. Eighty-seven percent of these patients were female. In 74 percent of these cases, the sexual contact between the psychiatrist and the patient included genital contact; in the remaining cases, the sexual contact consisted of kissing, fondling, and/or undressing. Other characteristics of the most recent patient contact are presented in Table 2.

Table 2. Characteristics of Respondents' Most Recent Sexual Relationship with a Patient

Characteristic	n	Percentage
Who initiated relationship ($n = 82$)		
Psychiatrist	9	11.0
Patient	26	31.7
Both	47	57.3
Length of relationship ($n = 84$)		
One sexual encounter	16	19.0
Less than 3 months	22	26.2
3–11 months	14	16.7
1–5 years	18	21.4
More than 5 years	14	16.7
Current status of relationship ($n = 83$)		
No contact whatsoever	37	44.6
Continued therapeutic contact, no sexual contact	3	3.6
Continued sexual contact, no therapeutic contact	6	7.2
Continued therapeutic and sexual contact	2	2.4
Married or in a committed relationship	11	13.3
Friendship, no sexual contact	24	28.9

Note. The total number of responses for each question varied because some respondents did not answer all questions.

Seventy-three percent of the offenders indicated that they engaged in the sexual contact for "love" or "pleasure." Nineteen percent intended the contact to enhance the patient's self-esteem and/or to provide a restitutive emotional experience for the patient. Other reasons for becoming sexually involved with patients included "loss of control," "exploitation," "judgment lapse," "impulsivity," "therapist enhancement," and "personal needs." Sixty-five percent of the offenders stated that they had been in love with the patient; 92 percent believed that the patients were in love with them.

In responses that were not mutually exclusive, offenders believed that the patients experienced the sexual contact as caring in 50 cases, helpful in 29, and therapeutic in 9, as opposed to exploitative in 11, harmful in 8, and inappropriate in 5. Overall, 25 percent of the offenders were pleased to have had this sexual contact, 35 percent had mixed feelings, and 40 percent regretted the contact. A larger percentage of the female offenders (50 percent) than of the male offenders (38.9 percent) regretted the sexual contact, but this difference did not approach statistical significance. The one-time offenders did not differ from the repeat offenders in their overall assessment of the contact.

When multiple responses were permitted, 18 percent of the offenders reported the use of sexual contact as a therapeutic intervention during treatment sessions, 17 percent indicated that it took place concurrent with therapy but outside of treatment sessions, and 69 percent stated that it occurred after termination. When the sexual contact occurred only after termination (in 63 percent of the cases), it was initiated within the first 6 months in 18 percent. We compared the respondents who initiated the sexual contact only after termination with the remaining offenders on all variables; there were no differences between these two groups in demographic characteristics, in whether there were repeat offenses, or in the status of the current relationship. The repeat offender (a 58-year-old married, board-certified American Psychiatric Association member) who acknowledged involvement with 12 patients was a member of the posttermination group. He reported that the most recent sexual contact began within days of termination, that he was in love with the patient, and that he was still sexually involved with the patient at the time he completed the questionnaire (although he was married to another woman). The only differences that emerged in a comparison of the pre- and posttermination groups involved the offenders' overall feelings about the most recent patient contact. Eighty-one percent of those in the posttermination group, as opposed to 41.4 percent in the pretermination group, reported that they were in love with the patient ($\chi^2 = 13.4$, df = 1, p < .001). Likewise, those in the posttermination group were less likely to regret the contact ($\chi^2 = 10.5$, df = 2, p < .01).

Forty-one percent of the offenders consulted colleagues because of their sexual involvement with patients. Repeat offenders were less likely to seek consultation than one-time offenders (22.2 versus 50 percent; $\chi^2 = 5.8$, df = 1, p < .02). Seventy-five percent of the female offenders consulted colleagues about their sexual contacts, as contrasted with 37.5 percent of the male offenders, but this difference was only marginally significant (Fisher's exact test, p = .0596, two-tailed). There were no other significant associations between the gender of the responder and response to the most recent sexual contact.

Psychiatrists' Sexual Contact with Their Own Therapists

Twenty (1.6 percent) of 1,233 respondents indicated that they had been sexually involved with their own therapist or analyst. Included in these 20 were 2 men who also acknowledged sexual involvement with their own patients. Female psychiatrists (n = 11, 4.4 percent) were more likely than male psychiatrists (n = 9, 0.9 percent) to have had sexual contact with a therapist (Fisher's exact test, p < .001, two-tailed). When multiple responses were permitted, 16 of the involved psychiatrists described the sexual contact as exploitative, 14 as harmful, and 10 as inappropriate, whereas 5 described it as helpful, 4 as caring, and 1 as therapeutic.

DISCUSSION

Although the return rate (26 percent) for the questionnaire might appear to limit the validity of our conclusions, several factors increase the probability that they are reliable. The 6.4 percent overall prevalence of psychiatrist-patient sexual contact in this survey is consistent with the prevalence of therapist-patient sexual contact reported in previous surveys of psychiatrists (Kardener et al. 1973) and psychologists (Holroyd and Brodsky 1977; Pope et al. 1979) that had considerably higher return rates (46–70 percent). Also, the gender distribution of our respondents is nearly identical to that of the population of psychiatrists in the United States from which the sample was selected. Two attributes of the respondent sample differed significantly from the total population of psychiatrists. First, respondents were slightly, although significantly, younger than those in the 1983 AMA Masterfile. As indicated in Table 1, the age differences are not marked, but with large samples, differences of small practical importance can give rise to statistically significant test results. A more noteworthy result is that 57 percent of the respondents were board certified, compared with 49 percent of those in the 1983 AMA Masterfile. This discrepancy suggests that board-certified psychiatrists were more likely to respond, possibly because they are more concerned about the issues or about the reputation of the psychiatric profession. The overrepresentation of board-certified psychiatrists should not invalidate the conclusions of this report, whereas underrepresentation might have led to charges of bias toward less skilled practitioners.

We assume that our data can provide only conservative estimates of the prevalence of psychiatrist-patient sexual contact. Some offenders are undoubtedly so concerned about confidentiality, despite assurances of anonymity, that they would never return a questionnaire of this nature. Furthermore, the 6.4 percent prevalence is not an accurate estimate of the number of involved patients, since many offenders are repeaters. It is also unlikely that the prevalence is inflated by false positives (i.e., claims of sexual contact that had not occurred).

The gender differences of the respondents are consistent with our hypothesis. Male psychiatrists were more likely than female psychiatrists to have engaged in single and repeat offenses, and the majority of patients involved were female. Furthermore, female psychiatrists were more likely than male psychiatrists to have been sexually involved with their own therapists.

In most cases the sexual involvement began during treatment or within 6 months of termination. A small minority of these cases resulted in committed relationships or marriage.

The majority of the offenders acknowledged that they engaged in sexual contact with patients for their own sexual or emotional gratification. These offenders were apparently unaware of, or willing to ignore, the clinical contraindications and ethical prohibitions (AMA 1985; Bouhoutsos et al. 1983; Edelstein 1943). They also believed that patients with whom they were involved had predominantly positive feelings about the sexual contact. Their assessments contrast sharply with the reports of our psychiatrist respondents who had been sexually involved with their own therapists, and with other reports in the literature (Bouhoutsos et al. 1983). The majority of the psychiatrists in our survey who had been sexually involved with their own therapists rated the experience as exploitative and harmful. Also, as indicated earlier, 90 percent of the patients in the Bouhoutsos et al. (1983) study were reported to have experienced negative effects. In another study, Feldman-Summers and Jones (1984) interviewed women who had been sexually involved with their therapists and compared them with a control group of female patients. They found that therapist-patient sexual contact produced a greater mistrust of men and therapists and a greater number of psychological and psychosomatic symptoms after the cessation of treatment.

Despite these studies (Bouhoutsos et al. 1983; Feldman-Summers and Jones 1984) documenting psychological damage to patients who have been sexually involved with their therapists, there is evidence that offenders tend to minimize the impact of their actions. Bouhoutsos et al. (1983) found that psychologists who had been sexually involved with their own patients could not realistically assess the effect of therapist-patient sexual contact on other patients. The offenders in our survey may also have had a distorted view of the effects on their own patients. Increased attention in residency training programs and continuing medical education courses to the consequences of psychiatric sexual abuse is clearly indicated.

Our finding that only 41 percent of the offenders sought consultation because of their sexual involvement with patients is nearly identical to that in another study, in which 40 percent of 20 involved psychiatrists and psychologists turned to their colleagues for assistance (Butler 1975). Although a smaller percentage of offending psychiatrists (33.3 percent) in our study were repeaters than the percentage of offending psychologists (80 percent) in Holroyd and Brodsky's study (1977), the relatively infrequent use of consultation by repeaters in our survey is disturbing. Are these psychiatrists unaware of the clinical and ethical contraindications? Are they sociopaths who have little concern for their patients and simply hope to avoid apprehension? Or are they expressing symptoms of other psychiatric impairment through sexual contacts with multiple patients? Further research into the psychodynamics of these offenders may help to clarify some of these questions.

We did not substantiate our hypothesis that single offenders would be more regretful about their sexual contacts than repeat offenders. Single offenders differed from repeaters only in the greater probability of their seeking consultation because of sexual contact. The absence of any other differences between these two groups of offenders may relate to the fact that we do not know how many one-time offenders are likely to become repeaters in the future.

Completing an accredited psychiatric residency clearly does not protect against subsequent sexual contact with patients. Although 87 percent of all respondents had completed accredited residencies, offenders were more likely than nonoffenders to be residency graduates. Furthermore, nine offenders became sexually involved with patients while they were psychiatric residents. Since sexual involvement with a patient would undoubtedly result in expulsion from a training program, involved residents may have been reluctant to discuss their behavior with supervisors. Rieker and Carmen (1983) noted that residents in their training program rarely discussed sexual countertransference feelings during supervision. Our data also suggest that residency training programs may be deficient in educating residents about psychiatric ethics and/or countertransference conflicts.

In conclusion, the findings of this study demonstrate that psychiatrist-patient sexual contacts continue to occur despite ethical and clinical prohibitions. The study also suggests that residency training curricula should be expanded to include specific educational programs on sexual abuse by psychiatrists. Furthermore, our data indicate that offenders may need encouragement to seek professional consultation and that patients may need assistance in coping with the negative consequences of involvement with therapists. We hope that subsequent investigations will provide additional information that will assist us in developing more effective means of preventing this unethical behavior.

Chapter 2

Sex Between Patient and Therapist: Psychology's Data and Response

Annette M. Brodsky, Ph.D.

Psychologists have been actively collecting data from colleagues, patients, licensing boards, and ethics committees on issues of sexual intimacies between patient and therapist. While the Chapter 1 survey on psychiatrists is the state of the art regarding the practice in 1986 of that population of subjects, there also exists a rather extensive history of data collection on the prevalence and incidence of this kind of misbehavior within the field of psychology.

Early references to the issue of sex between therapist and patient date back to the Hippocratic oath, which warns physicians not to have sex with their patients, and further back to statements in the code of the Nigerian medicine men, who were advised not to "sex the patient." The issue was discussed during the early days of psychoanalysis, particularly in a letter from Freud to Ferenczi (as cited by Jones 1957) suggesting that analysts who do not stop before a kiss might encourage other colleagues to go further: "There is no revolutionary who is not driven out of the field by a still more radical one" (p. 164). He noted that younger colleagues "will find it hard to stop at the point intended" (p. 164). Helene Deutsch (1944), on the other hand, took the position of denial of professional vulnerability in focusing on patients' "farfetched allegations," which she saw as "wish-fulfilling fantasies."

In the 1950s and 1960s, it is known that some professionals actually collected data on sex between patients and therapists, but feared formal presentation or publication of the results. Only in the 1980s was Forer encouraged to present his data, collected in the 1960s, on the frequency of this practice (Forer 1980). In 1955, Bruno Klopfer, a renowned psychologist, told his participants at an American Psychological Association Postdoctoral Institute about survey data he had collected in California, but did not formally communicate to the professional community regarding a "surprisingly large percentage" of psychologists and psychiatrists who had sexual contacts with patients (M. Gluck, personal communication, February 22, 1988). Dahlberg (1970) reported on his failed attempts to present a paper on the subject to a "larger organization," only to be told that the topic was too controversial.

Sex between patient and therapist was not clearly stated as unethical by the mental health professions until the mid-1970s. During the late 1960s and early 1970s two professionals published accounts of positive consequences and recommendations for therapist-patient sex. James McCartney (1966) wrote about "overt transference" as a visible, audible, or tangible muscular or glandular reaction to an inner feeling of a patient that represented a need to do more than talk. He got consent from patients and their families for having sex with patients. Martin Shepard (1971) wrote a book, *The Love Treatment,* suggesting beneficial effects of a therapist having sex with a patient. Both of these authors were widely read, and they provoked intense feelings about such practices. Both authors were psychiatrists and were negatively sanctioned by their professions.

In 1970, at the American Psychological Association Convention, Phyllis Chesler, a New York psychologist, presented her dissertation results based on a study of women's experiences of having sexual relationships with their therapists. She later wrote about the phenomenon (Chesler 1972a, 1972b) in conjunction with issues concerning the abuses of women in psychotherapy and other mental health treatments. Meanwhile, on another front, in 1970 Masters and Johnson published *Human Sexual Inadequacy,* which reported on women who had been sexually abused and exploited by previous health care professionals. They recommended stricter sanctions against such therapists and declined to use sex surrogates because of the potential for abuse (Masters and Johnson 1976).

Also, in the early 1970s, the first large awards for malpractice because of therapist-patient sex surfaced, with the most media attention being given to the case of the New York psychiatrist, Renatus

Hartogs, brought to court by his patient, Julie Roy. The case resulted in a $350,000 award for damages, which was later reduced considerably on appeal. The case became part of a cause célèbre, and the popular book *Betrayal* (Freeman and Roy 1976), written by the patient, was later made into a television movie.

In 1973 a task force on sex bias and sex role stereotyping in psychotherapeutic practices was formed by the Board of Professional Affairs of the American Psychological Association. This task force, chaired by the author and Jean Holroyd, had a mission to look at various ways that sex roles influenced psychotherapy, including sexual contact between therapist and patient. It became obvious that sexual seduction by therapists was a primary problem identified by respondents to its survey of practitioners (American Psychological Association 1975). When the task force asked the American Psychological Association Ethics Committee for the extent of complaints registered against psychologists for sexual contact, only four such complaints were found during the years 1970–1974. The worst sanction resulting from any of these cases was the removal from membership of one of them—for nonpayment of dues.

In the next decade, there would be over 100 cases brought to the ethics committee with complaints of sexual intimacies. A similar rise in cases reported to state licensing boards in psychology and other mental health professions occurred, and the increase in malpractice cases defended by insurers of mental health professionals would result in the American Psychological Association being dropped by one of its insurers, primarily on this issue. Today, sexual intimacy complaints represent the greatest number of malpractice claims against psychologists and the largest percentage of money used by insurers of any category for defending and paying judgments against psychologists (Bennett 1987). Currently, insurers have set a cap of $25,000 for defense and will not pay damages in a judgment against a psychologist for sexual intimacy with a patient.

Parallel to the awakening of the mental health professions, particularly psychology, about the problem of therapist-patient sex, was a focus on examining the incidence among practitioners. Based on results of the American Psychological Association Task Force on Sex Bias survey of psychologists who indicated a concern about sex between therapist and patient, Holroyd and Brodsky (1977) surveyed a random sample of 1,000 licensed psychologists in the 50 states regarding their "erotic practices" with patients. Responses were received from 70 percent of the sample, with the results indicating that 5.5 percent of the males and 0.6 percent of females admitted having engaged in sexual intercourse with their patients. Ten percent of males and 1 percent of females admitted to erotic practices, not necessarily including sexual intercourse. Of those who did admit having such erotic practices, 80 percent engaged in the behavior more than once, even though a frequent comment by those erotic practitioners was that it was not beneficial, but rather harmful to the patient and therapist alike.

This study was not the first survey of practitioners. It was based on a previous study by Kardener et al. (1973), who surveyed 445 male medical practitioners in Los Angeles and found 12 percent of male psychiatrists admitting sexual intimacies with patients. Perry (1976) later reported on a survey of 500 women physicians (of which 156 constituted the final usable data) in which none reported having sexual intercourse with patients, but many believed in and engaged in nonerotic touching. In another report, Holroyd and Brodsky (1980) found that the "erotic practitioners" of their earlier sample were more at risk for having sexual intimacies with patients, not if they used nonerotic touching, but only if the practice of touching patients was selective (i.e., one sex only). Pope et al. in 1979 surveyed members of the psychotherapy division of the American Psychological Association in the context of a survey regarding sex between educators and students. Their data were in line with the earlier studies—the overall incidence of sex with clients was 7 percent. In a 1986 mail survey of psychologists in private practice (Pope et al. 1986), 6.5 percent of the respondents admitted sexual contact with clients. In the most recent survey of psychologists (Pope et al. 1987), which focused on a variety of ethical practices and beliefs, only 1.9 percent of the subjects reported such contact. This striking decrease in incidence is graphically illustrated in Table 1.

Table 1. Studies of Therapist-Client Sexual Intimacy Incidence Among Psychologists

Date	Authors	Return Rate	Overall Incidence	Males	Females
1977	Holroyd and Brodsky	70%	7.7%	12.1%	2.6%
1979	Pope et al.	48%	7.0%	12.0%	3.0%
1986	Pope et al.	59%	6.5%	9.4%	2.5%
1987[a]	Pope et al.	46%	1.9%	3.6%	0.5%

Note. Values are percentages.

[a] Although the data were not separated by practitioner sex in the published article, personal communication with K. Pope (February 22, 1988) revealed these figures.

Explanations for the difference would be speculative, but factors to consider would range from the increasing awareness on the part of mental health professionals and consumers due to the press reports about malpractice cases, to the education and clearer sanctions by the professions, and to the recent legislative successes in criminalizing sexual misconduct between therapists and patients in some states. There may seem to be an imbalance in that more cases are being brought forth today at the same time that practitioners appear to be reporting less involvement, but one should bear in mind that the cases currently being reported are based on actions that may have been performed years earlier. Not only does the justice system tend to work slowly, but the patient's awareness of the unethical and illegal nature of the behavior often surfaces years later. The patient may need additional time to work with another therapist to come to a state of readiness to take any action against a therapist. Thus, the appearance of an increase in unethical behavior in this area, as opposed to a potential actual decrease of incidence in the therapeutic professions, may be a reporting lag.

The California State Psychological Association formed a task force on the issue of sex between patient and therapist, which surveyed California psychologists (Bouhoutsos et al. 1983). Based on a 16 percent return rate, the survey results were compatible with results of earlier studies of physicians and psychologists in previous surveys. The California task force surveyed therapists regarding information they had about patients who had had sex with former therapists. Ninety-two percent of the sexual relationships with former therapists reported by their patients were between male therapists and female patients. The majority (79 percent) of the former therapists were in private practice. The mean age was 42 years for the involved therapist and 30 years for the patient. The task force also reported on the damages therapists saw in patients as a result of having a sexual relationship with a therapist. Some results included: increased depression, loss of motivation, impaired social adjustment, suicidal intent, and increased substance abuse. Sequelae also included hospitalization, worsening of intimate relationships, and mistrust of the opposite sex and of therapists.

During the late 1970s and the 1980s many other researchers explored the nature of sex between therapist and patient. Studies ranged from small sample interview studies of patients or therapists to cross-sectional studies of other populations of therapists from many disciplines. The small sample of data tends to corroborate that of the large surveys. One can see the emergence of a typical picture of the kind of therapist who engages in sexual intimacies with patients, the rationales presented for the behavior, and the lack of remorse. Butler and Zelen (1977), from their interviews of 20 psychologists and psychiatrists who had sex with patients, found that the therapists tended to be vulnerable and needy. The sex was not planned and was not seen in hindsight as therapeutic for either the patient or the therapist. The therapists did not seek help, nor did they seem to be discouraged by their professions from continuing to have further alliances with patients.

The next section presents a composite of the data sources as they fit together into descriptions of the therapists involved, their patients, and attempts at sanctioning and rehabilitation. In addition to the above (and other) research studies on sexual intimacies, I have also drawn on my own experience from working with ethics committees, malpractice lawyers, licensing board investigations, and direct patient referrals to expand upon the statistically researched data with some impressionistic data of the information about relationships too small in incidence to be available statistically from random sampling of practitioners.

THE THERAPIST DESCRIPTIONS

What are the characteristics of the offenders? First of all, the therapist involved in sexual intimacy with patients is usually male. Most of the cases reported to ethics committees and licensing boards and in civil litigation are by women who are bringing cases against their male therapists. There have been female therapists involved as perpetrators, but most often these cases have been with lesbian patients and represent a small proportion of the total. Very few male-male dyads are reported. We know that intimacy between homosexual patients and therapists does exist, but they are not often represented in the ethics committees or the surveys. Those few that are known to researchers and sanctioning boards tend to be between adult males and their minor male patients.

The next variable is age. The modal therapist sexually involved with a patient is middle-aged, and he is typically about 16 years older than the patient. Younger male-female dyads appear to result from inexperience and naïveté of the therapist. Sometimes these alliances have led to marriage or a long-term relationship. It is only when this relationship sours and the woman realizes that the relationship was not based on a mutual level of consent at the beginning, but instead on the therapist's unfair use of knowledge of the patient's vulnerabilities, that a complaint may surface.

The older male therapist who becomes involved sexually with his patient is usually an individual who is involved in unsatisfactory love relationships in his own life. He may be in the process of going through a divorce, having had several marriages already, or he may have a history of poor relationships with women on the staff of the agencies in which he works. He tends to see predominantly female patients in his practice, and he is likely to be involved sexually with more than one patient at a time. These therapists are likely to treat patients differentially according to sex. That is, a male therapist who touches, holds, kisses, or hugs his female patients, but not his male patients, is at higher risk for sexual intimacy with female patients.

Another related aspect is the crossing of other boundaries important to psychotherapeutic practice. The therapist who becomes involved sexually with a patient is likely also to be a therapist who has patients work for him, or advise him in real estate or finances. The erotic practitioner may believe that because he is superior to other therapists, he is competent to go beyond the standard practices of his profession. He may feel that he can perform "innovative" techniques or be involved in extratherapeutic relationships with his patients, or that he is able to help patients whom other therapists are reluctant to see. He may be seen as a charismatic guru by his patients and by some students. Perhaps it is his many years of psychotherapy experience, but he is often too confident in himself and not inclined to seek help or consultation or even to communicate with other therapists about his cases.

A frequently reported behavior of therapists who become sexually involved with patients is that they inappropriately self-disclose to their patients. Many patients who have brought complaints can document knowledge of the marital and family problems, job conflicts, and other personal details in the lives of their therapists. Sometimes they have actually been taken by their therapists to professional conventions and otherwise treated as personal friends or family. The very fact that a patient knows much about the personal life of the therapist is an indication that professional boundaries have been crossed and that this therapist is now at high risk for sexual intimacy.

A personal characteristic of the sexualizing or erotic practitioner is that he is an isolated professional. Even if he works in a group practice or an agency, he does not closely consult with his peers.

Having been in practice for many years, he may have a good reputation in the psychological community. He is often a "good old boy." His colleagues do not really know what goes on in his therapy, and those who find out do not want to acknowledge this fact, even though, for example, the American Psychological Association ethics code enjoins a psychologist to bring unethical behavior to the attention of the offender as a first step in resolution. There is some indication from our knowledge of clinical cases that therapists who engage in sexual practices with their patients may spawn new generations of therapists who are likely to imitate this behavior. Boards and committees sometimes get complaints about therapists who have been trained by therapists who are known to have been sexually intimate with patients (see Chapter 13).

Physically, the therapists do not seem to have much in common, although they appear to have an aura of power or charisma in the eyes of the patient. The therapist may be perceived as distinguished looking, attractive, fatherly, or as emanating a certain warmth or power. Apparently, any of these characteristics may be enough for some of the patients to develop strong, early erotic transferences. As described by the patients, the sexual alliance itself may be very poor, but the patients are much more invested in the love aspect and the maintenance of the relationship than in the sex. In some cases it is the patient who takes on the role of being the therapist in attempting to help or console the sexually deficient therapist. The fact that she is needed for his growth and psychological well-being may be exactly what is so enticing to her. Because of confidentiality, it is very difficult to get information directly from accused therapists, although there have been some case studies and some small sample data on the dynamics of offenders, who may be quite immature (Rozsnafszky 1979) or who may have a masochistic desire to get caught (see Chapter 5).

THE PATIENT DESCRIPTIONS

The patients who are likely to become at risk for having sex with their therapists can also be identified by certain demographic and psychological characteristics. The patient at risk is most likely to be female. A homosexual patient of either sex with a same-sex therapist who is homosexual is the next most likely at risk. The patient is frequently reasonably attractive, young, naïve, dependent, and needs to work on relationships, particularly love relationships. Most patients who become sexually involved with their therapists do not enter therapy with presenting complaints about their sexuality. Sexual difficulties are often suggested or interpreted by the therapist as a problem area. The patients try hard to trust the therapist, even if they do not easily trust other people in their lives. The patients may or may not be sexually attracted to the therapist. If they are, this may be based upon their confusion of sexual feelings for the therapist with awe or love. By the time the sexual relationship is imminent, some patients are so invested in the transference relationship that whether or not they participate sexually is far less important to them than whether the doctor approves of them and that he does not abandon them.

Patients generally do not question the therapist's judgment when sexual intimacies are proposed or acted out. Rather, patients question their own judgment if it conflicts with the therapist's demands. If patients are not sexually aroused, they may hide this "deficit." When the therapist's behavior is identified to them later as being unethical and the therapist as having exploited them, these patients can feel devastated at their own inability to have recognized this earlier. Patients who become involved sexually with their therapist may have extremely high intelligence and may be in extremely responsible positions and happy marriages. It may be difficult for them to explain to family, colleagues, or others how they could have been so naïve about therapy.

One major group or type of vulnerable patients includes those who have been physically or sexually abused as a child. These patients may play out the abused child role with the therapist and may be very vulnerable to the therapist's demands. Reactions to the sexual intimacies vary with particular individuals, but a large number of previously abused (and also many who were never before abused or exploited) report out-of-body experiences or other related dissociative mechanisms during the sexual episodes. This is similar to what physical or sexual abuse victims have reported as a way of coping with their early childhood abuses. Patients who have not been sexually abused previously have also reported this type of reaction. They try to isolate the sexual experience, disown it, and take the rest of the therapy hour for what they can get.

According to the California Task Force Report on Sexual Intimacy (Bouhoutsos et al. 1983), which surveyed second therapists, 30 percent of the patients had had sex in the first few sessions. Later onsets of the first occurrence were reported with decreasing frequency down to a low of 4 percent within 3 months after ending therapy. The sooner sexual intimacy between therapist and patient began, the shorter the period of time that therapy could be sustained.

Consequences for patients included suicidal feelings or behavior and increased drug or alcohol use. Some were hospitalized and a few committed suicide. Other negative effects included worsening of sexual, marital, or intimate relationships; mistrust of the opposite sex; and adverse impact on marriages and/or families. Patients were suspicious and mistrustful of future therapists and love relationships, and some would not return to a professional for further help. The more intense the involvement, the greater the likelihood that the patients would not soon return to therapy to seek help.

REPORTING SEXUAL MISCONDUCT

That there is an increase in reporting this behavior is unquestioned. In 1973 when the American Psychological Association Task Force on Sex Bias requested its ethics committee to examine sexual intimacy cases in its files, only four complaints were filed between 1970 and 1974. Between 1974 and 1980 over 100 cases were filed, and since 1980 the single greatest category of cases brought to the ethics committee has been for sex between therapist and patient (Ethics Committee 1986). A parallel phenomenon occurs with licensing boards in the various states, such that increasing numbers of therapists are being brought to the attention of licensing boards and increasing numbers are losing their licenses for this behavior (Gottlieb et al. 1986). In general, there appear to be lower dismissal rates each year for sexual intimacy cases, which may suggest a trend of increasing stringency by both ethics committees and state boards. About one-half of the patients who have been involved sexually with their therapists expressed no awareness that it was unacceptable either ethically or legally. Also, a persistent 4-5 percent of therapists still report that sexual conduct between patient and therapist is not unethical (Pope 1987).

The American Psychological Association's Committee on Women has prepared a document for consumers that identifies the unethical behaviors of therapists who invite sexual intimacies and guides the patient through the choices of grievance avenues. This document is intended to be kept in offices of practitioners and in agencies, and to be made available to the media (American Psychological Association 1987). Consumer groups have begun around the country to help patients in posttherapy groups (such as the one at UCLA), or in recovery groups that are self-help (such as one developed by Sylvia Diamond in Texas). Professional agencies, such as the walk-in clinic in Minnesota run by Gary Schoener and his colleagues (Schoener et al. 1981), provide consultation as well as treatment and support. Their development of a mediation model for resolving mis-communications in cases in which patients and therapist are still willing to come to a rapprochement after a sexual intimacy has occurred is perhaps the most encouraging step for rehabilitation (Bouhoutsos and Brodsky 1985; Schoener 1986).

Unfortunately, there is no specific data as yet on the long-term effects of supervised rehabilitation of therapists who have had sex with patients. It is known that there are cases where such rehabilita-tion will not work. Poor candidates are those therapists who have been discovered to have had sex with more than one therapy patient, who show no remorse, and who do not believe that sexual intimacy can harm patients; in particular they are those about whom patients made complaints of sexual overtures during the therapists' supposed re-habilitation period. As mental health professionals, we have an obliga-tion to protect the public. There are therapists who probably never should have been licensed in the first place. We do not have very good data on our failures at keeping inappropriate practitioners from be-coming licensed. We are moving in the direction of criterion-based licensure and behavioral rehabilitation, but we have a long way to go. Hence, our work is cut out for us. We need prevention, better screen-ing of applicants in training programs, and training of new therapists in ways of avoiding involvement in the first place.

Chapter 3

Sexual Contact Between Social Workers and Their Clients

Lucille Gechtman, M.S.W., L.C.S.W.

Among the major mental health professions, social work is a late-comer in addressing the problem of sex between its members and their clients. Data on the incidence of sex between psychiatrists and their patients were first published in 1973 (Kardener et al.). Although the initial survey of psychologists was first done in the late 1960s (Forer 1980), the first published account of psychologist-patient sex, using Kardener et al. as a model, was in 1977 (Holroyd and Brodsky). The attention to this issue in social work journals is scant, and no survey of social worker–client sex has yet been published. This void is an ironic contrast to the historical view of social workers as moral agents of society (Siporin 1982).

In an effort to lift the veil of secrecy surrounding social worker–client sex, and to spur the profession into joining the fields of psychiatry and psychology in first acknowledging, and then addressing this problem in a serious and systematic manner, this author joined with a noted researcher of therapist-patient sex and completed the first national survey of social workers in 1985 (Gechtman and Bouhoutsos).

This chapter will present some of the important findings of that survey, discuss the apparent lower incidence among social workers, and comment on the social work profession's relative lack of interest in investigating this area.

METHOD

In July 1984 a random selection of 500 male and 500 female members of the National Association of Social Workers (NASW) was mailed a one-page, 18-item confidential questionnaire. At the time of the survey, NASW membership was approximately 97,450. The questionnaire essentially followed the format of the Kardener et al. (1973) and Holroyd and Brodsky (1977) studies but contained additional items including the gender of the clients with whom they were sexually involved, sex after termination of treatment, whether they had been in therapy, other social work professionals with whom they were sexually involved, the type of social work degree, licenses and certification, and whether their social work curricula contained material about attraction and/or sexual involvement with clients. The respondents were asked if they believed that erotic contact between social worker and client could under certain circumstances be beneficial to clients. Social workers were also asked if they ever seriously considered having erotic contact with a client, and given the right situation, would they engage in erotic practices with their therapist, client, or student? They were asked if they had ever engaged in the following activities with a client: erotic kissing, erotic fondling or petting, oral-genital stimulation of or by the client, or sexual intercourse, and whether these activities took place during the therapy session, during the course of therapy, or within 3 months or beyond 3 months after termination. Respondents were asked whether they had engaged in erotic activities with a social work teacher, supervisor, administrator, employer, student, supervisee, employee, or their own therapist. Additionally, they were questioned about nonerotic hugging, kissing, or touching.

RETURN AND DEMOGRAPHIC INFORMATION

The only identifying information noted from the returned questionnaires was the date and state or country on the postmark. No differences were found between early and late responders. The return rate was 54 percent, a generally acceptable rate for this type of survey.

The respondents ranged in age from 28 to 85 years, with a mean of 50 years. There was no significant difference in the return rate by gender (51 percent women, 49 percent men), but the sample included more younger men (48 years or less) and more older women (49 years or more).

The percentage of Masters of Social Work (M.S.W.) degree holders in our sample (88 percent) was the same as the general NASW membership. However, 11 percent of the sample held doctorates (D.S.W. or Ph.D.), compared to 5 percent for NASW. Fifty percent stated that they had had some personal therapy. Overall, 54 percent of the respondents reported that they used nonerotic contact with male or female clients.

The subject of sexual involvement with clients had been addressed in the social work training programs of 14 percent, and sexual attraction to clients had been addressed in the programs of 33 percent. States that licensed social workers provided 59 percent of the respondents, and 54 percent of the respondents were licensed. Incidentally, at the time of the study, 38 states licensed social workers; currently 44 offer licenses to social workers.

EROTIC CONTACT WITH CLIENTS: ATTITUDES

Erotic contact was defined in this study as one or more of the following activities: erotic kissing, erotic fondling or petting, oral-genital stimulation of or by clients, and sexual intercourse.

The overwhelming majority of respondents (90 percent) stated that they believed that erotic contact between therapist and client could not be considered beneficial under any circumstance. Eight percent were unsure. Only 2 percent thought that it could be beneficial. Five percent indicated that they had seriously considered engaging in erotic contact with a client if the "right situation presented itself." There was a significant gender difference in these responses. Twenty-four male social workers and 1 female social worker responded that they had seriously considered erotic contact with a client.

In response to the open-ended invitation to write comments about the study, 9 respondents expressed anger at the researchers: "The suggestion of erotic involvement with the client is so unprofessional I don't want to share in the survey"; "It is because of people like you that social workers have such a poor reputation with the general public"; and, "I will not dignify this study with a response." Other respondents expressed disbelief and shame: "I am so ashamed of social workers who engage in erotic experiences with their clients that

I have dropped my professional practice and am exploring new careers." And, "If the time has arrived where this information need be asked of social workers, then it might be time for me to cease functioning under this label." Twenty comments expressed gratitude for the interest and research in this area. Several doubted whether those who had engaged in erotic behavior with their clients would answer honestly. Fifty-six comments (11 percent) emphasized disapproval of erotic contact with clients and described it as sick, exploitative, acting out, confusing to clients, contaminating the treatment, a gross violation of trust, or taking advantage of clients' vulnerability.

EROTIC CONTACT WITH CLIENTS: PRACTICES

Erotic contact during the course of therapy was reported by 1.3 percent of the respondents. Erotic contact with clients only after termination of the therapy was reported by another 0.6 percent. Sexual intercourse during the course of therapy was reported by 1.0 percent and only after termination by another 0.1 percent. All 10 of these respondents were male. Overall, the survey revealed that 3.8 percent of male social workers had erotic contact with clients during the course of therapy and/or after termination of therapy.

Seven of the 10 had erotic contact during the course of treatment; 3 only after termination. Six had sexual contact during the treatment sessions themselves. Of the 4 who did not engage in sexual intercourse, 2 participated in erotic kissing, 1 in oral-genital stimulation of the client, and 1 in oral-genital stimulation both of and by the client. This group of 10 used significantly more nonerotic touching than social workers who were not erotically involved.

Seven of those involved in erotic contact were involved only with opposite-sex clients; 2 only with same-sex clients; and 1 was involved with both male and female clients.

At the time of the survey these 10 respondents ranged in age from 32 to 65, with a mean of 49. We did not learn what age they were at the time of the sexual involvement.

All 10 had at least an M.S.W. degree; 2 had Ph.D.'s (compared with 5 percent of NASW membership). They received their graduate degrees between 1953 and 1978. The social work curricula of 4 of the 10 contained material about attraction to clients but only 1 had instruction related to sexual involvement with clients. No significant relationship was found between the type of degree and whether or not they learned about therapist-client attraction or sex in their social work education.

Seven of the 10 had fulfilled additional requirements for inclusion in the National Academy of Certified Social Workers (compared with 54 percent of NASW membership). Six were licensed in states that offered licenses; 2 who were unlicensed came from states that did not license social workers; and only 1 had no license in a licensing state. No significant relationship was found between erotic contact and state licensure or national certification.

Two of the 10 believed that erotic contact with clients could, under certain circumstances, be beneficial; 6 did not believe that assertion, and 2 were unsure. Six (compared with 34 percent of the total sample) wrote additional comments on the survey form. Four expressed regrets. One indicated that he would only become similarly involved again after the termination of the professional relationship. The 6th insisted that he had never participated for his own pleasure, but only to help the client feel accepted when he responded to "client initiated" erotic activity. Of the remaining 4 men who made no comments, 3 had been sexually involved with male clients.

Five of the 10 had been in personal therapy for from 1 to 5 years. One-half had had no therapy at all. For the total sample, there was no significant association between personal therapy and erotic involvement with clients.

In reaction to several commenters' belief that therapist-client sex was a California phenomenon, the location on the postmark was noted. Two of the responses came from California (Los Angeles and San Bernardino), while one each came from Arizona, Utah, Michigan, Missouri, Maryland, North Carolina, and West Virginia.

SEX IN OTHER PROFESSIONAL SOCIAL WORK RELATIONSHIPS

The respondents reported that 3.6 percent of them engaged in erotic activities with their social work supervisees, 1.9 percent with their social work students, 2.7 percent with their social work employees, 0.6 percent with their social work teachers, 1.3 percent with their social work supervisors, 1.0 percent with their social work administrators, 1.1 percent with their social work employers, and 0.6 percent with their own therapists. Only female respondents, 3 of them, reported sexual involvement with their own therapists. The 10 respondents who were sexually active with clients reported significantly more sexual involvement in these other dual professional relationships; 3 were sexually involved with social work students, 2 with social work employers, 1 with a social work clinical supervisor, 1 with a social work teacher, 1 with a social work employee, and 1 with a social work administrator.

Comparison of Social Work with Psychiatry and Psychology

Comparing the percentages of social workers with the different studies of psychiatrists and psychologists must be done with caution. The years in which the studies were conducted, the sample selection, the array of questions on the form, whether the study was local or national, the return rates, whether posttermination sex was included in the figures, and other such factors may influence the findings and their interpretations.

As these are initial data for social work they provide only tentative findings that are in need of replication. However, the social work figures are consistent with an incidental finding from a 1975 study of social workers focusing on attitudes and use of body and sex therapies, which indicated that 1.8 percent of the respondents used sexual intercourse and 10.8 percent approved of the use of sexual intercourse between the social worker and client for the purpose of sex therapy (Schultz 1975). As indicated in Chapters 1 and 2, the figures for psychiatrists and psychologists have been fairly consistent across all studies (Gartrell et al. 1986; Pope et al. 1979, 1986).

Our national survey of social workers revealed that 2.6 percent of the male social workers and none of the female social workers were involved sexually with their clients during the course of therapy. The studies on which this survey was modeled indicated that 10 percent of male psychiatrists engaged in erotic behavior, apparently during treatment (Kardener et al. 1973), and 10.9 percent of male and 1.9 percent of female psychologists had erotic contact with their patients during the course of treatment (Holroyd and Brodsky 1977).

The ratio of female to male social workers is approximately three to one; this ratio is reversed in psychiatry and psychology. Given that the sexually involved therapist is usually male, the incidence of therapist-client sex in the social work profession as a whole is much less than our survey figures indicate.

Why the Lower Incidence?

Social work has always been predominantly a woman's profession. It developed in the tenth century among middle-class women who formed organizations to combat the hardships of industrialization and urbanization. The impetus came in part from evangelical Protestantism, which was identified with Christian piety, moral integrity, compassion, self-sacrifice, maternal concern, and its belief in the moral superiority of women (Rhodes 1985). The "responsibility mode," described by Gilligan (1982) and applied to social work by Rhodes, refers to the female voice, which focuses on caring, responsibility, and nurturance in accordance with people's needs. This "responsibility mode" is seen as embodying many of the basic ideals of social work practice.

The men in social work would be more likely through self-selection, training, and professional identity to possess more of the traditional female characteristics of caring, responsibility, and sensitivity to the needs of others. It may be that these attributes are incompatible with sexual exploitation of clients, that the essentially oral nature of social work precludes genital involvement with the objects of nurturance.

More social workers, compared with the other major mental health professionals, practice in institutional or agency settings. The 1985 NASW Data Bank National Summary Tables reveal that a variety of agencies provide the primary employment setting of 89 percent of its members (compared to 14 percent of psychologists); 11 percent are in private practice only, and 56 percent have private practice as their secondary employment setting. The initial psychology survey done in 1968 (Forer 1980) found just a single instance of sexual involvement with patients on the part of psychologists practicing in institutions, and a 1983 study of psychologists (Bouhoutsos et al.) found that only 14 percent of reported cases of therapist-patient sex occurred in institutions. Agencies and institutions do offer less privacy, more time accountability, and therefore less opportunity than private practice for sexual involvement with clients. Agencies are likely to establish clear boundaries between social worker and client. Furthermore, the support system provided by an institution, including supervision, contact with colleagues, case conferences, and in-service training, are apt to deter those at risk from engaging in inappropriate behavior with clients.

The lower incidence might in part be a product of less honesty in admitting to the sexual activities on the questionnaire as those behaviors could be felt to be too dissonant with professional social work values. Might power, class, or status differentials between social workers and their clients, and between social workers and psychologists and psychiatrists contribute to sexual distancing? There is no firm evidence as yet to endorse these possibilities.

SOCIAL WORK'S LACK OF INTEREST IN EXPLORING SOCIAL WORKER-CLIENT SEX

During the past decade, there has been increasing attention given to the subject of therapist-patient/client sex. Numerous theoretical papers, empirical studies, and surveys have been published in journals of psychology, psychiatry, and psychotherapy. It is hard to find an annual meeting of the American Psychological Association or the American Psychiatric Association that does not have papers, symposia, and workshops devoted to this issue.

There is an impressive body of research and systematic analysis concerning the harm that results from therapist-patient/client sex (Bouhoutsos et al. 1983; Chesler 1972a, 1972b; Durré 1980; Sonne et al. 1985). Juries are assessing the damage done to clients as so great that NASW's malpractice insurance carried, in early 1985, coverage limited to $25,000 inclusive of legal fees for offenses involving sexual misconduct.

The lay public is exposed to discussion of therapist-client sex on television news, talk shows, and specials. The harmful effects on clients and the violations of professional ethical codes and sometimes of criminal laws are broadcast in many publications read by the general public.

Complaints against social workers have increased. The national NASW office reports that between 1955 and 1977 there were 8 complaints against its members, compared with 18 complaints in the period between 1980 and 1985. Locally, the California Board of Behavioral Science Examiners indicates that between July 1982 and December 1983 there were no complaints, between January 1984 and October 1985 there were 7 complaints, and between November 1985 and November 1987 there were 15 complaints filed against social workers for sexual practices with clients.

In spite of the attention being given to therapist-client sex, a review of the social work literature including the fall of 1987 reveals only several articles related to this subject (Brown 1985; Gareffa and Neff 1974; Holtzman 1984; Schultz 1975; Shor and Sanville 1974). No survey of social worker–client sex has yet been published. The first and to date only national study of sexual contact between social workers and their clients, completed in 1985 and reported in this chapter, has not been granted acceptance by the leading social work journal. This study had an acceptable return rate (54 percent) and used a survey form, methods for selecting a sample, a sample size, and techniques for statistical analysis and inference that were comparable to published studies of psychiatrists and psychologists. Since the coauthor has been sole author or coauthor of a number of works in the area of therapist-client sex, the rejection is not likely to be attributable to lack of knowledge base or the writing style of the manuscript.

The paper based on this survey of social workers, presented in October 1985 at the annual meeting of the California Society for Clinical Social Work, the California Institute for Clinical Social Work, and the National Federation of Societies for Clinical Social Work, was placed last in a 2-day program, was poorly attended, and evoked no later inquiries.

Social work was also later than the other major mental health professions to include specific prohibitions against sex with clients in its formal ethical code. Whereas, in the 1970s, both the American Psychiatric Association and the American Psychological Association published explicit prohibitions against sex with patients, it was not until 1980 that the prohibition, "the social worker should under no circumstances engage in sexual activities with clients," was written into the NASW Code of Ethics (NASW 1980).

There have been some scattered social work efforts to address the problem. For example, the Minnesota Chapter of NASW, assuming an active role in this area, is involved with a walk-in counseling center that assists clients who feel they have been abused by their therapists. In the case of accusations against social workers, the chapter is aggressive in pursuing investigations. The Wisconsin Chapter of NASW worked for a bill that was signed into law in 1984 that imposed misdemeanor penalties on psychotherapists found guilty of engaging in sexual contact with their patients or clients. The national NASW News has occasionally printed articles condemning social worker–client sex (State punishes 1984; "Sexploitation" 1985).

Lack of interest involves more than resistance to the subject. It should be recognized that social work has a mission that is broader than that of many of the other helping professions. Clinical issues have to compete for the attention and resources of social work with the wide range of social concerns involving the health and welfare of the larger society and related political action.

However, the failure of the social work profession to address the existence of therapist-client sex within its ranks appears in part to be related to major changes that have recently taken place in social work moral philosophy. Max Siporin (1982) is one of the few voices in social work urging the profession to face this subject and to publicly debate these issues. He identifies a shift from a concern with ethical matters in traditional, normative terms to nonnormative libertarian moral and ethical positions and speaks of the social worker's desire to be impartial and not impose his or her personal values on clients.

One theory offers an explanation for the lack of written materials about sexual transference issues in a predominantly woman's profession by addressing the difference in the way male and female therapists handle the sexual feelings of patients (Moteki 1987). Female therapists must always be vigilant about not stimulating sexual advances from male patients as the female is perceived to be the inviter of sexual attention unless she specifically indicates she is not. Because sexual attraction is not usually addressed in training, the problem is felt by each female clinician to be personal and too intimate to be translated into professional literature.

Comments from the respondents to the social work survey provide some additional clues about the resistance of the social work profession. Quoted earlier in the chapter, some comments revealed an inability to deal with distasteful information as seen by the reactions of shame, denial, disbelief, self-righteousness, and blaming.

Minimizing the problem because only a small percentage of social workers is involved is another attitude that contributed to the failure to investigate this issue. A highly critical reviewer of our study wrote, "Isn't the point that a significant proportion of social workers aren't having sex with their clients?"

DISCUSSION AND CONCLUSION

Although social work is tardy in recognizing and addressing sexual contact between its members and their clients, reluctance to explore this taboo area is not limited to social work. Resistance experienced by the early psychology researchers is documented by Dahlberg (1971), and Davidson (1977) similarly speaks of the "problem with no name" for the field of psychiatry. Our survey of social worker–client sexual contact, providing the initial data for social workers, can open the door to the full attention that is presently given to this issue in the fields of psychology and psychiatry.

Social workers may experience an initial reaction of pride from the results of this study, which indicate that their violations appear to be less than those in the other major mental health professions. But this response must be tempered by the fact that a number of our colleagues are exploiting their clients, and others are at risk for doing so. It is a matter of concern that the findings of this study suggest that 1 of 10 social workers believes that under certain circumstances sex between therapist and client can be beneficial (2 percent) or is unsure if it can be beneficial (8 percent).

Increasing numbers of social workers are practicing privately because of reduced public funding of social programs. Many recent social work students are seeking M.S.W.'s as a route to becoming psychotherapists in private practice, with little commitment to social work's mission, distinctive functions, and dual focus on the individual and society (Rubin and Johnson 1984). If these trends continue, it is likely that social work violations will increase.

There were several areas emerging from the social worker study that require further discussion and clarification: social worker–client sex after termination of treatment, sexual involvement in other social work professional relationships, and nonerotic contact with clients.

There is no explicit mention in the social work ethical standards about sexual contact with clients after termination. Comments from the social work survey reveal that some social workers believe that sex between therapists and clients after termination of treatment is acceptable behavior. A review of the literature leads to the conclusion that termination does not eliminate the harmful consequences of therapist-client sex (Pope and Bouhoutsos 1986).

Social work is without formal guidelines regarding sexual intimacies in the context of other social work professional relationships. The social work survey found that 6 of the 10 social workers who engaged in sex with their clients also had sexualized other professional relationships, a significantly higher proportion than the remainder of the respondents. Sexualizing of professional relationships may be seen as being symptomatic of a more general inability to maintain clear and appropriate professional roles and boundaries.

There is confusion about the conditions under which nonerotic touching may be ethical, appropriate, and therapeutic. In the survey of social workers, a majority (54 percent) of the respondents employed nonerotic touching. Those who were sexually involved with their clients reported significantly more nonerotic contact with their clients than was reported by their colleagues. These findings contrast with a previous study, which found that under certain circumstances erotic practitioners were less likely to engage in nonerotic touching than were nonerotic practitioners (Holroyd and Brodsky 1977). The value of touching is acknowledged by Borenzweig (1983), who found that one-half of the clinical social workers in his study touched their clients, 83 percent had a positive attitude toward touching clients, and most believed that they were capable of separating affectional and clinically oriented touching from sexual contact. However, a traditional viewpoint holds that touching of any kind is never appropriate. As one of the respondents to the social work survey remarked, "We were taught to keep the desk between the client and therapist."

An unexpected and distressing finding of the social work survey is that education, licensure and certification, and therapy are not effective in preventing social worker–client sex. What then can be done to address the attitudes and behaviors that culminate in social worker–client sex?

The profession is urged to provide leadership in acknowledging this issue as a problem and to break through the defensive postures that prevent its resolution. It must provide leadership in articulating formal ethical, clinical, and professional standards of conduct that address therapist-client sex comprehensively, forcefully, and unambiguously. Social work conventions and journals should welcome and encourage theory, research, and vigorous discussion of this phenomenon. Schools of social work, field placements, textbooks, licensing procedures, and the whole panoply of formal and informal means for ensuring ethical and efficient behavior on the part of all social workers should be engaged in dealing honestly and openly with this topic.

Social work must put its house in order, regardless of the fact that the disorder is apparently less than in other mental health professions. It should be entirely unacceptable that anyone practicing under the aegis of social work should violate the special trust given the profession and harm any of those whom social workers are empowered to help.

Chapter 4

Therapist-Patient Sex Syndrome: A Guide for Attorneys and Subsequent Therapists to Assessing Damage

Kenneth S. Pope, Ph.D.

Every one of the major mental health professions has formally and explicitly banned sexual relations between therapist and patient. Therapist-patient sexual intimacies have led to multimillion dollar malpractice judgments and to therapists losing both their membership in professional organizations and their license to practice as a professional. About one-third of the states have passed laws declaring therapist-patient sexual intimacy to be illegal, thus eliminating the need for expert testimony to establish that this act violates the standard of care. Prominent clinicians (e.g., Masters and Johnson 1976; Redlich 1977) have urged that health care professionals who engage in sex with their patients be charged with criminal or statutory rape. At least one state (Wisconsin) holds sexual intercourse between therapist and patient to be a Class D felony.

Taken together, these facts reflect with dramatic clarity the immense harm that therapists inflict when they engage in sexual relations with a patient. So great is the damage that the ethical prohibition is ancient and absolute, and the penalties are forceful.

Systematic research and case studies have documented the destructive effects of therapist-patient sexual intimacies (Bouhoutsos et al. 1983; Burgess 1981; Butler 1975; Chesler 1972a, 1972b;

D'Addario 1977; Feldman-Summers and Jones 1984; Freeman and Roy 1976; Plasil 1985; Pope and Bouhoutsos 1986; Stone 1980; Vinson 1984; Walker and Young 1986). In her review of the evidence to date, Durré (1980) found that "amatory and sexual interaction between client and therapist . . . is detrimental if not devastating to the client" (p. 243).

Clinicians must educate themselves about the major aspects of harm that therapist-patient sex causes. First, this education can help clinicians to understand the rationale for and to observe without exception the absolute prohibition against therapist-patient sexual intimacies. Second, it will enable them to recognize the symptoms in their own patients who have been sexually intimate with a previous therapist. The research suggests that over one-half of all therapists will treat such patients (Pope and Bouhoutsos 1986). Third, it demonstrates the need for clinicians to work effectively in their professional organizations to enforce the ban on this harmful activity and to develop strategies of prevention.

Attorneys likewise must understand the damage caused by therapist-patient sexual involvement. Without such understanding, they may not fully recognize that such behavior is an inexcusable tort. Moreover, they may find it difficult to establish an effective working relationship with potential clients.

THERAPIST-PATIENT SEX SYNDROME

The sequelae to therapist-patient sexual intimacy may form a distinct clinical syndrome, with acute, delayed, and chronic aspects, to which I have applied the term *therapist-patient sex syndrome*. There are at least 10 major damaging aspects of this syndrome.

Ambivalence. Perhaps no aspect of therapist-patient sex syndrome tends to be so demoralizing for the patient—and occasionally for the subsequent therapist—as the patient's ambivalent feelings about the exploitative therapist. The phenomenon is similar to the experience of many survivors of child or spouse abuse: At times the individual fears, despises, and wishes to escape at all costs from the abusing authority figure; at other times, the individual feels close to and wishes to cling to, take care of, and even protect the abuser. Occasionally, the individual may experience both sets of feelings simultaneously.

One source of this intense ambivalence is the intense attachment that therapists allow or urge patients to form. Patients involved in a sexualized therapy often describe their therapists as if they were parental (or in some cases, godlike) figures. A deep, primitive attachment forms, of the sort an infant or very young child might develop toward a parent. Therapists are viewed as omniscient and omnipotent providers of essential care. Patients, therefore, respond with feelings of intense gratitude and dependency.

Exploitative therapists can be extremely adept at creating, nurturing, and reinforcing such exaggerated and irrational attachments. Even when patients begin to realize that they have been exploited and can intellectually understand the damage that the sexualized therapy and therapist have caused them, these primitive feelings tend to remain until they are finally worked through.

Many times, the feelings toward the exploitative therapist have been overlaid or "grafted" onto the actual early childhood feelings of patients. Such patients may experience the therapist as if he or she were the actual parent. Even if only on a "feeling" level, patients may experience any negative reactions toward the exploitative therapist as if they constituted an abandonment of, betrayal of, and attack on the actual parent.

Thus, once the damaging effects of the sexualized relationship begin to occur, patients may feel caught in an intolerable yet inescapable trap: On the one hand, they sense that the therapist has harmed them and will tend to cause ever greater—perhaps fatal—harm; on the other hand, any attempt to remove themselves from this destructive relationship and process seems a dangerous (in light of the seeming omnipotence of the therapist) and disloyal (as if one were betraying a beloved parent) act.

Working through this Gordian knot of ambivalent feelings and impulses in a subsequent therapy tends to be a long and difficult process. Part of the problem is that the subsequent therapy itself may be experienced by patients as betraying the parental figure of the prior therapist.

Guilt. The sense that patients are betraying a powerful, caregiving, parental figure—discussed in the previous section—can be part of the guilt induced by therapist-patient sexual intimacy. But the more fundamental and chronic guilt feelings involve patients' sense of responsibility for the sexual involvement. They become convinced that they—not the therapist—were in control of the therapeutic sessions and therefore brought about the sexual contact.

This irrational guilt is similar to that experienced by many rape and incest survivors. The rape survivor, for example, may be tortured by a variety of relentless self-criticisms: "If only I had dressed differently." "Why didn't I struggle more?" "Couldn't I have chosen a different route home?" The rape survivor has trouble grasping the fact that the rape is the responsibility of the rapist, not of the person raped. Similarly, incest perpetrators may dwell—in their attempts at self-justification—on the supposed "seductive" nature, words, or acts of the incest survivor; and incest survivors—even long into their adult years—may blame themselves.

Therapy patients often find it very difficult to work through these persistent feelings of guilt. Both they and the exploitative therapists who attempt to blame the victim to escape legal and ethical accountability forget that it is always and without exception the therapist's responsibility to ensure that no sexual intimacy occurs.

One complicating problem is that patients often experience intense positive transference that may involve sexual attraction to the therapist, may at times dress or act in a manner that some would characterize as "seductive," and may in fact experience difficulty in handling sexual impulses. But this no more justifies a therapist engaging in sexual relations with such patients than an adult's form of dress justifies rape or a child's seductive manner justifies incest.

In many cases, sexual issues and concerns may have prompted individuals to seek therapy in the first place. But in all cases the therapist must recognize and handle in a professional manner patients' dependence and vulnerability, the power differential, and the phenomenon of transference. When therapist-patient sexual intimacy occurs, it is never the fault of the patient.

Emptiness and isolation. So pervasive are the sequelae of therapist-patient sexual intimacy that they seem to affect the very sense of self, particularly of the self in relation to others. Patients who have been sexually involved with a therapist often attribute such power and significance to the therapist that they feel empty or "unreal" unless they can be "filled up" through the direct sexual involvement. They feel alone and isolated unless connected—literally—to the therapist. Even long after the sexual involvement has ceased, such patients—like many incest survivors, rape survivors, and battered children or spouses—may feel as if they were absolutely alone in their ordeal, as if they had been somehow singled out by fate for this unique torture. For this reason, reading the accounts of other patients who have been sexually involved with a therapist and taking advantage of chances to talk and share experiences, either formally through group therapy or through some informal channels, with other patients may be an important part of subsequent recovery.

Sexual confusion. Sexual intimacies with a therapist are likely to leave patients extremely confused about their own sexual nature, sensations, impulses, and experiences. Even if sexual issues were not part of the presenting complaint, exploitative therapists tend to create and utilize patients' sexual confusion. Some patients may want to be held—physically but nonsexually; unprincipled therapists may relabel this as a desire for sexual union, or at least use the initial physical contact as a pretext for sexual contact. Other patients may desire to use therapy to work on such issues as low self-esteem, a lack of fulfilling interpersonal relationships, a desire for more spontaneity, or burnout. In all such instances, therapists may either redefine the problem as fundamentally sexual in nature or present a sexual solution to what seems to be a nonsexual problem. Such comments might include: "Your low self-esteem is due to your inability to be in touch with, accept, and appreciate your body." "Your interpersonal relationships are unfulfilling because you have trouble acknowledging and expressing the sexual aspects." "You lack spontaneity because you inhibit your sexual impulses." Or, "Your feelings of burnout are due to a blockage of your sexual energies."

If such rationales seem strained and hard to accept, it is probably because it is so easy to forget how desperate many people are when they begin therapy and the degree to which they must place great trust in the therapist. Sexually exploitative therapists can be quite adept at playing upon patients' insecurities, dependence, trust, and transference.

Impaired ability to trust. This consequence of therapist-patient sexual contact is clear, unmistakable, and completely understandable. Patients place great trust in their therapists. They often discuss taboo subjects, think aloud about the "unthinkable," and may tell their therapists secrets known to nobody else. They can come to feel a basic trust akin to what an infant develops for a parent.

When this trust is violated, the patient's ability to establish or accept a trusting relationship or to feel trust itself may be badly damaged, perhaps permanently impaired. For this reason, many patients who have been sexually intimate with a therapist are unable to participate in any subsequent therapy. Moreover, many have difficulty trusting an attorney, a medical doctor, or any other professional or person in authority.

Identity and role reversal.   In this area, therapist-patient sexual intimacy again reveals a similarity to incest. In incestuous families, the child often seems to become "the parent" of the actual parent. In this reversal of roles and identities, the child seems oriented to, and in some cases extremely skilled at, taking care of the parent. The child becomes attuned to the needs of the parent, not only in the sexual realm. This, of course, is a perverse and destructive reversal of the parent-child relationship.

So too in a sexualized therapy, the patient may become the "therapist" to the therapist. Many patients have noted that the sexualization of the therapy began gradually, with the therapist beginning to talk about himself or herself. Soon the focus of therapy became the therapist's rather than the patient's problems. And an underlying, if not more blatant, theme of the therapy became the patient taking care of the therapist's needs, sometimes not only sexually but also emotionally, clerically, financially, and in a variety of other ways.

Emotional lability or dyscontrol.   Patients who have been sexually intimate with their therapists often feel baffled by and at the mercy of a chaotic surge of conflicting emotions. Their emotions can be intense and unpredictable. Laughter may give way suddenly to an out-of-control sobbing. The lack of emotional stability can aggravate these patients' general sense of insecurity and can be extremely demoralizing and confusing. During a subsequent therapy, just when they feel that they have their feet on the ground and have achieved some emotional balance, they can—seemingly without warning—plunge into a profound depression.

Suppressed rage.   Like the survivors of incest, rape, or battering, patients who have been sexually exploited by their therapists may develop a deep and powerful rage but be unable, for long periods of time, to act upon, to talk about, or sometimes even to acknowledge this reaction. The ambivalence, the role reversal, and the guilt described above all make it very difficult for patients to acknowledge and accept, let alone take action in regard to, the anger that is a natural and understandable reaction to such betrayal, exploitation, and harm. Moreover, exploitative therapists tend to deflect criticism or anger, teaching patients to turn such negative impulses inward.

Increased suicidal risk.   Subsequent therapists and attorneys need to maintain alertness to any signs that patients who have been sexually involved with their former therapists may be suicidal, for increased suicidal risk is common. The suicidal impulses may come from a variety of sources. They may be a result of the suppressed rage toward the exploitative therapist which patients may turn inward against themselves. The impulses also may be the patients' way of expiating the irrational sense of guilt or they may be what seems to patients the only way to respond to the double bind associated with the ambivalence. Suicidal impulses may be an expression of the hopelessness felt by the patients, hopelessness about ever being able to reach out to any source of help that would address the intolerable feelings of emptiness and isolation.

Cognitive dysfunction.   Therapist-patient sexual intimacy seems to exert particularly destructive effects on cognitive functioning. The most frequent impairment is in the area of attention and concentration, often involving flashbacks, intrusive thoughts, unbidden images, and nightmares. This psychological dysfunction can make it impossible for some patients to carry out the most simple and routine daily tasks. In their most extreme state, such cognitions bring memories (related to the exploitative therapist and sexualized therapy) into awareness with the intensity and immediacy of events happening in present time. In this area, therapist-patient sex syndrome bears similarities to posttraumatic stress disorder.

WHY CLINICIANS AND ATTORNEYS MAY FAIL TO RECOGNIZE THERAPIST-PATIENT SEX SYNDROME

Despite the devastating effects of therapist-patient sexual intimacies, the patient's need for subsequent clinical services, and the patient's right to legal representation, clinicians and attorneys alike may overlook, deny, misinterpret, minimize, or in comparable ways fail to acknowledge and respond adequately to the patient's plight. The reasons patients may find subsequent therapists and attorneys nonresponsive to their situation are numerous.

Ignorance that therapist-patient sex is wrong. This lack of knowledge has become less common as the phenomenon of therapist-patient sex has received more publicity. And yet some attorneys—and occasionally clinicians—are apparently unaware that therapist-patient sex is inappropriate. Attorneys who are not knowledgeable in this area may view sex between therapists and patients as simply sex between two consenting adults, and therefore without specifically negative consequences. Comparison might be made to sex between, say, a grocery store owner and customer, a homeowner and gardener, or a physical fitness instructor and client. Such attorneys may ask rhetorically, "What's so special about sex between therapists and patients?"

Ignorance that the mental health professions have prohibited therapist-patient sex. Even if attorneys—again, who are not specialists in this area—concede that therapist-patient sex is inappropriate, they may believe that such a case would be difficult to win if they are unaware that there is an explicit standard of care that prohibits the act.

Narrow preconceptions about the occurrence of therapist-patient sex. Clinicians and attorneys alike may fail to recognize therapist-patient sex if it fails to meet certain preconceptions. For example, most of the literature on the subject refers to male therapists and female patients, but therapist-patient sex occurs not only in the other three possible dyads but also in triads and larger groups. Other preconceptions may involve specific conditions, for instance that the therapist uses threats, force, or intimidation. Yet the routes by which therapists become sexually involved with their patients are diverse. The following list—taken from Pope and Bouhoutsos (1986) and used with permission—presents the 10 most common scenarios:

1. Role Trading: Therapist becomes the "patient" and the wants and needs of the therapist become the focus.
2. Sex Therapy: Therapist fraudulently presents therapist-patient sexual intimacy as a valid treatment for sexual or other kinds of difficulties.
3. As If . . . : Therapist treats positive transference as if it were not the result of the therapeutic situation.
4. Svengali: Therapist creates and exploits an exaggerated dependence on the part of the patient.
5. Drugs: Therapist uses cocaine, alcohol, or other drugs as part of the seduction.

6. Rape: Therapist uses physical force, threats, and/or intimidation.
7. True Love: Therapist uses rationalizations that attempt to discount the clinical/professional nature of the relationship with its attendant responsibilities.
8. It Just Got Out of Hand: Therapist fails to treat the emotional closeness that develops in therapy with sufficient attention, care, and respect.
9. Time Out: Therapist fails to acknowledge and take account of the fact that the therapeutic relationship does not cease to exist between scheduled sessions or outside the therapist's office.
10. Hold Me: Therapist exploits patient's desire for nonerotic physical contact and possible confusion between erotic and nonerotic contact. (p. 4)

Bizarreness of the episode. Some patients' accounts of their experiences with therapists (e.g., being treated literally like a dog) may be so peculiar that listeners reflexively dismiss the allegations. However, as with rape and incest, the bizarreness of the account per se is no simple guide to its veracity, one way or the other.

Misunderstanding informed consent. Consent is simply not relevant in the area of therapist-patient sexual intimacy, any more than it is in the area of incest. Aside from such facts that it is always the therapist's responsibility (rather than a "shared" responsibility in which the patient could ever contribute to the malpractice) to ensure that sexual intimacies never occur, or that consent to this act within the context of transference cannot be truly free and informed, is this fundamental concept: There can be no consent that legitimizes a clearly unethical and illegal act. The patient's "consenting to," "authorizing," "initiating," or "asking for" sexual relations with a therapist has no more meaning than a patient's consenting to, authorizing, initiating, or asking for a nonphysician to perform surgery or dispense illegal drugs.

Guilt. As discussed in a previous section, patients may carry with them a heavy burden of irrational guilt. They may see themselves as completely at fault, as "causing" the malpractice. Unprepared subsequent therapists and attorneys can unwittingly collude with such patients in this misattribution.

Apparent functioning. Some patients may be able to "hold themselves together" for long periods of time—sometimes years—

subsequent to the sexual involvement. The harm can evolve gradually beneath an extremely well-defended public persona. Defenses such as denial and repression serve to mask the damage from self and others. The syndrome can thus have a delayed aspect, similar to many cases of posttraumatic stress disorder. In such cases the damages are not readily apparent to subsequent clinicians and attorneys.

Attributing allegations to mental disorder. Some clinicians and attorneys alike may share an unfortunate tendency to attribute virtually all complaints patients voice against therapists to the psychopathology of the patient. Any dislike of a therapist must be attributable to "negative transference." Any claims against a therapist are dismissed as hallucinations or delusions.

However, the patient's presumed or actual psychopathology is never a valid reason to reflexively dismiss a patient's allegations of sexual involvement with a therapist. Patients suffering from the most severe forms of psychopathology may be most vulnerable to sexual exploitation.

Attributing damages to a preexisting condition. Clinicians and attorneys who are not knowledgeable in this area may be at risk for reflexively attributing a patient's current problems not to sexual intimacy with a therapist but rather to the preexisting problems that led the patient to seek help from the exploitative therapist. What seems to be the case, however, is that, aside from whatever separate problems are caused by the sexual involvement, two consequences related to the preexisting condition occur: (1) the sexualization of the therapy nullifies any genuine therapeutic effects and thus the patient is deprived of the timely treatment sought for the preexisting condition, and (2) the worse the patient's condition prior to the sexual involvement, the more pernicious the effects of the sexual involvement.

Continuing sexual involvement. Some clinicians or attorneys may dismiss a patient's claims of being harmed by sexual involvement with a therapist using the following reasoning: If the involvement actually took place or if it were actually harmful, the patient would never have returned for a second "session." They are incredulous about patients who have apparently remained for years within a sexual relationship with a therapist.

What this view does not take into account is the power differential between therapist and patient—the transference, dependence, reliance on authority, eagerness to please, confusion, and the numerous ploys, both physical and psychological, which therapists can use to exploit their patients. The psychological bondage that keeps many sexually exploited patients unable to break free from the therapist is similar to that which keeps battered spouses from leaving their marriages or incest survivors from leaving home.

The patient's anger, motivation, or style.   Patients may be so consumed by their anger that they have a hard time communicating clearly with subsequent therapists or attorneys. They may seem dominated by the desire for revenge, and thus come across as less than credible. They may have a difficult interpersonal style—perhaps related to formal psychopathology—that impairs their ability to form a rapport with someone or to tell their story in a coherent, persuasive manner. Unfortunately, the listener's primary response may be an urge to "get rid of" such patients as quickly as possible, generally by referring them elsewhere.

Inappropriate boundaries of therapy.   Attorneys and other nonclinicians may assume that therapist-patient sexual intimacies are legitimate if they do not happen at the therapist's office during the time that a session is scheduled. It is as if the therapeutic relationship—with all its attendant responsibilities—somehow dissolved outside the therapist's office or at times other than scheduled sessions. Sexual intimacies between therapists and patients are always unethical, regardless of where or when they occur.

Defensive pride in the profession.   Subsequent therapists may wish to ignore, minimize, or otherwise cover up their patients' accounts of sexual intimacies with previous therapists due to a false professional pride. They may believe that nothing should be done to bring discredit to the profession (especially if the consequent publicity should steer patients to another profession or should lead to additional regulatory measures by external organizations). They may use all the resources at their disposal to avoid airing dirty professional laundry in public.

Sympathy for a colleague.   Subsequent therapists may empathize with the therapist who was sexually involved with the patient. They may believe "there but for the grace of God go I." This impulse—in conjunction with the previous item—has led to the "conspiracy of silence" in which professionals refuse to acknowledge or take any action in regard to the malpractice of their colleagues. It is only recently that this self-interested denial of patient rights and well-being has begun to lessen. It has not, as yet, disappeared completely.

The Bad Samaritan.   Therapists—like any other humans—are vulnerable to the tendency to want to not become involved in difficult or messy situations. They may not want to become even indirectly involved with a licensing board or ethics committee if their patient files a formal complaint. They may fear a countersuit from the prior therapist. For these and similar reasons, they may overlook or minimize the patient's dysfunction or distress resulting from the relationship with the former therapist.

Sense of omniscience.   Attorneys and subsequent therapists may fail to conduct an adequate assessment of the patient's condition if they feel so certain of their knowledge (or ignorance) in this area that their instant and superficial judgment suffices. Listening to the patient tell his or her story while attempting to understand what happened is unnecessary in this atmosphere of arrogance; the attorneys and therapists presume to know all that needs to be known without taking the trouble to learn and understand.

Attraction to the harmed patient.   Subsequent therapists and attorneys may find it difficult to carry out their duties in a responsible and effective manner if they themselves feel sexually attracted to the patient. On one hand, they may let their professional obligations fall to the side while they attempt a subtle—or not so subtle—courtship. On the other hand, they may feel so threatened by their own feelings of attraction that they maintain an excessive psychological distance from the patient—they figuratively shove the patient away. In a recent national survey, 87 percent of therapists acknowledged feeling sexually attracted to at least some of their patients (Pope et al. 1986). Over one-half (63 percent) of these therapists reported that the attraction made them feel guilty, anxious, or confused. This discomfort with attraction may pose a barrier to an adequate assessment of the patient's condition and needs.

Bias.   Finally, attorneys and subsequent therapists may simply be biased against patients who have been sexually intimate with a prior therapist. In some instances, this bias may be associated with the therapists' or attorneys' own sexual behavior with patients or clients. For example, Holroyd and Bouhoutsos (1985) found that clinicians who had engaged in sexual intimacy with their patients were biased in their assessments of damage done to such patients, even if the patient assessed had been sexually intimate with another therapist rather than the one doing the assessment.

RESPONSIBILITIES OF SUBSEQUENT CLINICIANS CONDUCTING ASSESSMENTS OF THERAPIST-PATIENT SEX SYNDROME

Other chapters in this volume provide information about conducting therapy for patients who have been sexually intimate with former therapists. In this section, guidelines are presented for screening patients to identify those who have been sexually involved.

Be alert to the possibility with each patient. As the initial chapters in this volume indicate, sexual intimacies with patients continue despite the legal, ethical, and professional prohibitions. In light of evidence that up to 80 percent of these incidents are attributable to repeat offenders, a large number of patients have been and continue to be harmed. It is important to be aware of this possibility with any patient who has previously been in therapy. The guilt and associated aspects of therapist-patient sex syndrome may induce patients to conceal this prior involvement. Like many rape and incest survivors, they are ashamed of their history. Sensitivity to and respect for the patient's feelings about the prior involvement are crucial.

Listen carefully. Let patients tell their stories in their own way. Especially given the possible feelings of shame and guilt, patients need "breathing room." It is easy for us to project our own feelings and expectations onto the initial revelations. What is essential is to clarify what the patients actually experienced and how it affected them.

Provide for possible emergencies. One aspect of therapist-patient sex syndrome is increased suicidal risk. Particularly with a syndrome that shares many dynamics with posttraumatic stress disorder, the suicidal impulses may erupt suddenly. Ensure that self-destructive impulses are monitored carefully.

Don't practice law. In a situation in which there are numerous legal rights and needs, the clinician may be more than eager to offer well-meaning legal information, guidance, advice, and opinions. This will likely be a great disservice to the patient. It is, for the therapist, the practice of law without a license. A patient's suffering may be compounded by a clinician's attempt to play lawyer. In some cases, the stringent statutes of limitation may run out before the patient makes contact with an attorney. In other cases, the filing—and the timing of the filing—of formal complaints with licensing boards and ethics committees may drastically affect the prospects of a malpractice suit.

A useful simile involves the patient's medical needs. For a patient whose condition has clearly medical aspects, the therapist who attempts treatment without referral to a qualified physician risks charges of malpractice. Similarly, for a patient whose condition has clearly legal aspects, the therapist who attempts treatment without referral to a qualified attorney also puts himself or herself at risk.

Respect the patient's decisions.   Unless the state has a mandatory reporting law, it is always the patient's decision whether or not to file formal charges. Some clinicians may be so outraged at the previous therapist's behavior or so alarmed at the possibility that the previous therapist will harm other patients that they virtually demand that the patient file a complaint. Other clinicians may forcefully dissuade the patient from filing a complaint, perhaps because the therapist does not want to become involved in the proceedings, perhaps because the therapist does not feel that it is in the patient's best interests. The decision, however, like privilege, belongs to the patient rather than to the therapist.

GUIDELINES FOR ATTORNEYS REPRESENTING PATIENTS WHO HAVE BEEN SEXUALLY INTIMATE WITH A THERAPIST

Be aware of therapist-patient sex syndrome's implications, not only for the legal case, but also for your working relationship with your client.   Therapist-patient sex syndrome describes a person who is in pain and who experiences difficulty carrying out day-to-day tasks. These dysfunctions and distress may interfere with the client's ability to establish a smooth working relationship with an attorney. The patient will likely have difficulty trusting another authoritative professional. He or she may have trouble with attention and concentration, interfering with the ability to keep straight the various strands of a civil case or to remember appointments. Ambivalence and guilt may cause the individual constantly to change his or her mind about whether to pursue the case. To the degree that the attorney can understand that these and related phenomena may be sequelae of the sexual involvement, he or she may be better prepared to be genuinely helpful to the client.

Be aware of the common challenges. Defense attorneys tend to use fairly predictable techniques in challenging a patient's charges of sexual involvement and the resultant harm. The first line of defense is usually that the sexual involvement never occurred but rather was the result of: (1) the hallucinations or delusions of a very fragile patient who has impaired contact with reality, or (2) an attempt at revenge by a patient whose attempts to proposition the therapist were forcefully declined. Whether the sexual involvement actually occurred is a matter for the triers of fact.

If sexual involvement is established, the defense is often similar to that which has been customary in rape trials, for example, the patient initiated it, the patient enjoyed it, and the patient suffered no real harm. In addition, defense attorneys may attempt to delve into the sexual history of the patients and to present them in the worst possible light.

A final line of defense is that, even if the sexual contact occurred and may have been unwanted, nevertheless the patient's current dysfunction and distress are due to a preexisting condition. As mentioned earlier, it is likely that preexisting pathology or damage intensifies the harm resulting from sexual involvement with a therapist.

In anticipating these various challenges, what is crucial is that the attorney prepare the client. Such challenges may be psychologically devastating to a client who, for example, already feels deep guilt. Adequate preparation is absolutely necessary.

Be aware of fundamental sources of information. In order for the attorney to understand a client's current condition and the ways in which it has been affected by sexual relations with a therapist—and for the attorney to help a judge or jury understand these concepts—there are three major resources among the mental health professionals. First, there is the subsequent treating therapist. This clinician has worked with the patient over time, has seen him or her through crises, has heard more than once the patient's accounts of involvement with the prior therapist. It is this professional who will probably be able to provide the most vivid and detailed portrait of the patient.

Second, there is the clinician who conducts an extensive psychological and, if necessary, neuropsychological assessment. The clinician who gathers and presents this data serves three major functions: (1) the tests often seem more "scientific" to judges and juries than the testimony of even the most experienced and credentialed therapist; (2) this clinician can compare the current test results to any data (such as school records and previous testings) collected before or during the previous therapy; (3) because the clinician will almost certainly be spending less time with the patient than the current therapist and will be administering what are often perceived as objective tests, the clinician may be viewed as potentially less aligned with, less "on the side of" the patient.

Third, there is the expert witness who testifies that sexual involvement with patients is a violation of professional standards of care and that it causes damage, which can occur in the form of therapist-patient sex syndrome. This professional—because he or she has had no contact with the patient and has not carefully studied the chart notes of either the current or the previous therapist—is generally viewed by the judge and jury as even more disinterested. Both plaintiff and defense attorneys can elicit professional opinions that bear more directly on the case through the use of hypothetical questions.

These three separate professionals can help the attorney as well as the judge and jury understand the patient's condition and how it occurred. Each contributes his or her own unique content and perspective. Their professional observations and opinions supplement, of course, whatever testimony is provided by the patient and others, such as friends, neighbors, family, the clergy, or fellow workers, who can tell from a layperson's perspective and in a layperson's language how the patient was before the sexual involvement with the therapist and what has happened to the patient since that time.

CONCLUSION

Therapist-patient sex syndrome is a conceptual schema organizing the common sequelae of sexual involvement of patients with therapists. Like rape response syndrome and reaction to incest, it is probably underdiagnosed due to a variety of factors, many of which were discussed in a prior section. It is important for both clinicians and attorneys to understand the syndrome and to be alert for it in their patients or clients. If the diagnosis is missed, there is inadequate foundation for the professional services that follow. The diagnosis should be made, of course, only by a licensed clinician knowledgeable in this area of practice. Attorneys who find that their clients have been sexually involved with a therapist as well as therapists for whom assessment of this syndrome lies outside their realm of expertise should consider prompt referral to an appropriate clinician for a comprehensive examination. An adequate assessment of the sequelae of sexual intimacies with a therapist is crucially important not only for the formulation of a sound treatment plan or legal strategy but also for the establishment of a sensitive and understanding working relationship with the patient or client.

Chapter 5

The Seduction of the Female Patient

Sydney Smith, Ph.D.

The term *seduction* brings to mind the idea of inducing another person into sexual relations without the use of force or threat. The idea of being sexually seduced seems burdened with conflicting feelings: There is the excitement of finding oneself a desired sexual partner or a degree of pleasure in discovering that one can be the source of another person's sexual arousal. But there is also the fear or the moral prohibition or an inner concern that to allow oneself to be swept away in the charged atmosphere of the seduction itself may lead to dangerous outcomes such as abandonment or rejection or the fear that once the sexual needs of the seducer are satisfied, his interest will evaporate. Indeed, the fairy-tale longing that the seduction will culminate in a never-ending love is rarely realized.

The seduction of little children, on the other hand, has never been regarded as a genuine expression of love but, on the contrary, has been uniformly labeled as perversion, as taking advantage of the child's innocence, and thus in the efforts to protect children from such premature experience, the law has forbidden sexual relationships between adult and child.

This dichotomy leads into a central issue that arises today in the increasingly publicized sexual contacts between male psychotherapists and female patients. The layperson, upon hearing about such an encounter, looks upon the female patient as an adult who has the power within her possession to bring the seduction of the therapist to an abrupt end. As the defense lawyer expressed it in a recent legal case, "All she had to do was to get up and walk out." That comment casts the woman patient in the role of being totally in charge of her feelings, of being conscious of her own transference reactions, and of understanding fully the nefarious purpose of the treater. But the woman patient under these circumstances is seldom in control of any of these issues. What is more typical is that the woman patient is caught up in the throes of her own past, of her childlike feelings, of experiencing emotions that are powerful and frightening and that often lead the woman in such a posture to feel that she is at that moment not in charge of any aspect of her life. She is often at such times experiencing troubling reactions that take the form of confusion and fear and mixed emotions. She is thus led into a mesmerized state that precludes her from coming to terms realistically with what is happening.

In short, the woman patient at such moments is in a state of psychological regression—a retreat into a childhood state not only emotionally, but also intellectually. At that moment she becomes the helpless child again, reliving the experiences of the past, unable to cope with what is happening to her, feeling robbed of the ability to make choices, perceiving herself as small and weak and therefore unable to defend herself, hoping that whatever she is caught up in will represent an expression of love instead of the hate such patients remember from the past.

Women who find themselves in such a predicament usually come into treatment from one of two different historical sets of circumstances. First, there are women who have been sexually abused during childhood, usually by the father, and who have experienced strong sexual feelings—albeit infantile—for the father or some father-substitute. These fathers may have played out a mock seduction with the child in the sense of some kind of love play, but in many instances have had actual sexual contact with the child. Then the stage is set for the longings of the child to take on a powerful sexual significance, which then may be subtly introduced into later relationships with men, including the psychotherapist.

The sexual overtones introduced by the patient represent a reliving of the past and offer the therapist an important opportunity for interpreting this past and its accompanying needs and feelings, thus allowing the patient to discover her origins and bring about a separation between the infantile perception of father and present reality. In this way the patient can become free to make her own choices, and her insights into the nature of her childlike needs can be understood for what they are, allowing the patient to escape from the bondage of the past into a new freedom of choices. What one sees in such women initially is a form of dependence that can arouse in the therapist the recognition that this patient will comply with any action the therapist suggests in order to keep the loving father intact. As always in such instances the major therapeutic action is interpretation, but there are therapists who are in some way as needy as the patient and thus persuade the patient that her feelings are meant only for the therapist and that sexual contact with the therapist is a way of requiting the intense longings of the woman patient.

It is at this moment that much of the patient's mature intelligence seems to disappear, since typically what happens is that the patient becomes caught up in what she sees as a marvelous fulfillment of the infantile dream. What is also typical is that the therapist tires of this contact long before the patient, so ultimately the patient will be confronted with what can be a devastating rejection that then worsens whenever psychological issues may be involved. The next therapist has the task ahead of him or her made far more difficult by the mismanagement—indeed, the malpractice—of the earlier therapist.

The second set of circumstances involves a different scenario. Many women who come into treatment have suffered what they feel has been neglect. In their backgrounds, they were not as children convinced that they were loved or appreciated, and in their growing-up years, they have felt overlooked and sometimes ostracized with no conscious awareness of why they have had to suffer in this way. As a result of such childhood feelings, these women become convinced in later years that they are unattractive, that they are unlikely to find sexual fulfillment or be discovered by some man who would become the father and lover they never had. At some point, they enter treatment with a male therapist, hoping to overcome their chronic latent depression and discover some magical formula for improving their lives.

At the moment the woman patient enters therapy and begins to sense the special interest of her therapist—an interest that goes beyond the usual concern a doctor has for a patient—she is likely to respond with a sense of excitement. The idea that the therapist could see her as someone special, as an object of his love, suddenly becomes a powerful force in the patient's life, one that typically begins to take on all the attributes of an obsession. The patient begins to think of nothing else; her dreams are suddenly filled with the presence of the doctor and his comforting contact with her. Such dreams are not necessarily explicitly sexual, but they clearly indicate that the positive transference has been triggered in the patient.

Ordinarily these reactions need not be disturbing if the therapist is aware of what is going on. But if the therapist supports the patient's perception and colludes with her dreams (which he has been responsible in setting off), then both patient and therapist have launched themselves on a dangerous course, the consequences of which could be devastating for the patient. Any sense of moral prohibition in the patient is usually thrown to the winds, in part because the wish to be loved, and the more infantile wish to be cared for completely, begins to take charge of the patient's thoughts, and any concern about the inherent dangers in such a process is pushed to the further corners of the mind.

In either case, women patients caught up in such seductions in their treatment react differentially to the predictable rejection by the therapist. Some become angry, vindictive, and litigious, and seek redress through the courts. Others become weaker, more regressed, more isolated, and more difficult to reach, falling within the role of the victim and acting as if all hope must be abandoned. Indeed, these patients sometimes commit suicide. But there are also those who gather their strength and continue the search for the idealized father who, they are sure, will be embodied in the next therapist. For these women, the search must be continued, the effort renewed, the fulfillment further sought.

THE ABUSING THERAPIST

Further questions raise the issue of why the male therapist becomes caught up in acts of sexual abuse. Why does he risk his career, turn his back on his training, abandon the therapeutic task, and bring injury to another human being who is usually already too wounded to deal effectively with the betrayal of the therapeutic contract? The answers to these questions are not easy to find, because if the patient does nothing to stay the abuse or if she quietly leaves the therapeutic work, no one may know what agonies she has suffered or what was taking place between patient and treater.

But despite the lack of an opportunity to study such therapists at close range, it is not difficult to spell out at least a few of the issues that must be involved in cases of sexual abuse. First, abusing therapists demonstrate a great need for control. The therapist, therefore, must always be right, must keep the upper hand in conveying to the patient that he is all-knowing and all-powerful. The patient becomes the object first of a psychological subjugation that may, as the therapist grows bolder, become a form of physical subjugation. Such therapists enjoy a sense of triumph as they take custody of the patient's body as well as her mind. And the sense of control is even more prominent if the patient regresses to a state of the confused child and is therefore unable to understand clearly what is occurring or to what extent the patient's judgment and defenses have given in to the seduction.

Or in another scenario the therapist is not able to deal with his own psychological problems or with his own tensions, which leaves him vulnerable to finding his purpose in life too intertwined with his patients. He may have arrived at a point where it is necessary for him to hang on to his patients out of a profound need for reassurance and the development of some purpose in life. Under such circumstances these therapists usually abandon the psychotherapy processes to confide their personal problems to the patient, which may then arouse the patient to find ways to comfort the therapist, and this comfort can be quickly turned into sexual acts. In these cases, the woman may, through her misconceptions, assume the upper hand and become mentor to the therapist in a fashion that becomes intertwining and mutually dependent. Such relationships often end in the courts because the therapist tires of the interaction and the patient feels injured and betrayed.

The danger is always that the therapist under such conditions will use the treatment for his own ends rather than for the benefit of the patient, and, as a result, the therapy is corrupted and the patient's issues are set aside. One can often see how the therapist may overreact to the positive comments of the patient, not understanding the psychological meaning or manipulations lying behind such efforts on the part of the patient to make the interaction more personal. The therapist's need to feel important blinds him to the real significance of the patient's comments, and his response is to become expansive and all too often seductive in the presence of such women patients.

What such misuse of the therapeutic interaction reflects is the lack of attention given during the course of training to helping the would-be therapist to undo his errors, to develop the skills to stay on target, and to not find himself in a position of having to figure everything out for himself. The therapeutic task demands a good deal from the therapist if he is safeguarding the patient from his own issues. Often the therapeutic relationship becomes an extension of the relationships outside of therapy, thus becoming entangled in the needs of both patient and therapist, but where—also too often—the therapist's masculine wish for dominance overwhelms the female patient. When one hears what has gone on in the therapy hour, one is not confronted with a loving relationship, but more usually aggressive acting out on the part of the therapist that has little to do with the art of love.

There are those who blame such circumstances on the fact that the therapist may be suffering a lack of comfort in his private life. Usually this benign suggestion turns out to carry only a kernel of truth, since most cases that have come to light and have been studied are not instances of a genuine "falling in love," but are instead reflections of the psychopathological, egotistic needs of the therapist who abandons the well-being of the patient for his own crass self-indulgence. To try to give it a prettier formulation misses the importance of the sadistic character of such therapist-patient interactions.

With some therapists, it is clear that the act of sexual intercourse with a patient emerges out of the therapist's own castration anxiety. He is looking for reassurance on this issue. His sadistic treatment of the woman patient may well be an effort to defend himself or to find a defense against the anxiety by treating women abusively or by keeping the woman patient subjugated and exploited, thereby allowing himself to feel more whole. In certain cases such behavior toward female patients is stimulated by the transference. These patients take on the aura of the "bad woman," which in turn sets off the therapist's castration fears. In these cases, the therapist's seduction of the patient has nothing to do with love or caring or tenderness, but is an effort to keep the woman patient overwhelmed and controlled.

The therapist indeed may be attempting in his treatment of the female patient to cure his own mother. Something in the behavior or appearance of the patient may set off such reparative efforts. But this task also involves a good deal of gratification for the therapist—a kind of repetition turned back on itself, which allows the therapist to play out his own infantile needs while at the same time attempting to be the gratifying son.

Finally, there are therapists who engage in criminality out of a sense of guilt. Freud accidentally stumbled on this concept in hearing from patients how they would be overcome by guilt without knowing what the guilt was about. If they then engaged in some forbidden act, they experienced a sense of release because the guilt was at least attached to something. But the real guilt is connected to the male child's wish to murder the father and make mother into a sexual partner. This unconscious fantasy may not be so far removed from the therapist's wish to turn the patient's sexuality toward himself and replace the husband-father in the patient's life. This playing out of the fantasies of childhood seduction is far more common than is usually realized. The therapist brings these internal fantasies to bear on the patient's treatment, which turns out not to be curative for either patient or therapist, since the patient ends up being used for the therapist's purposes, and the therapist does not succeed in eliminating his own sense of badness, since the unconscious crime is only repeated and never resolved. Acting out this inner conflict never permits either a sense of completion or a fulfilling resolution. The underlying pathology drives the therapist back again to a repetition of his own problems.

THE REGRESSIVE SYNDROME

A major factor in what happens to the woman patient caught in the coils of a sexually abusing therapist is the arousal of a regressive self-image. It is as if the woman patient loses control over her own will as well as the dimensions of a powerful, controlling, parental figure who cannot be crossed or disobeyed. This return to an infantile state weakens the patient's resolve and leaves her with the conviction that she is a helpless figure, unable to overcome the strength of the treater or to escape his psychological hold on her. Old childhood fears reappear, and the idea of being abandoned by the therapist assumes awful proportions. Through the phenomenon of transference the therapist has been imbued with the magical capacities of the early father who is idolized or feared, or is the source of punishment and who has the power to discard the patient.

The reliving of childhood fears becomes painful and troubling, since in the regressed patient's mind, the only way to keep the father-figure around is by being obedient and undemanding; and if one has to suffer the ordeal of sexual abuse, that activity is the price of not being cast aside. How severe these reactions become in the patient depends on the severity of the child abuse at the hands of a punitive, frightening, or unloving parent. The question is always one of how much masochism is developed in a patient by a sadistic parent, which then sets the stage for a sadistic therapist. In such a situation the woman patient feels as if she has no choices and no way of defending herself, caught up as she is in the childhood hope that what is happening to her is an expression of love.

The element of regression in this process can move in two directions: The therapist becomes a sexual lover, but is cast in the role of the father, which deepens the patient's regressive state; or the therapist becomes increasingly sadistic, and the patient's regression goes over the edge into a depressive psychosis. Even when the patient falls into such a dreadful state, the therapist does not relent on his demands and thus jeopardizes the patient's life by driving her either into a deeper psychosis or into suicide. In some instances, therapists have been known to place the patient on two or three medications, adding further drugs as the "therapy" progresses, until the patient is taking a whole compendium of medicines. If and when the therapist becomes concerned about the nature of his contact with the patient being exposed, he then will abruptly remove all the medications, thus placing the patient in jeopardy of dying, since an abrupt withdrawal of multiple medications can have a lethal outcome. This approach to controlling the patient may be the ultimate expression of the therapist's sadism.

Yet, for the woman patient in these circumstances, it appears as if the therapist cannot be contradicted because, like father, he is all-powerful, and the attachment to the father-therapist is like that of the small child who reasons that negative attention is better than no attention at all. The sadistic therapist blames the patient for whatever goes wrong. The patient is reviled by the therapist on every front: She is told that she is ugly, that her wish for some kind of fulfillment is not merited, that her illness is an expression of her own badness, and that her sexuality is not exciting, and only out of her sexual neediness does the doctor have contact with her at all. Generally such abusing therapists keep the female patient dependent. These patients are locked into the relationship because they are convinced that no one else would put up with them, that their minds and bodies hold no interest, and that the ministrations of the therapist—sexual or otherwise—occur simply out of the goodness of his heart. The alternative is total abandonment, as if without the presence of the sadistic therapist, they would simply be left to die.

Thus, the woman patient's transference to the treater mirrors all of the therapist's reactions. She feels unloved and worthless and suffers from a continuing depression, seeing herself as helpless, small, and weak. The inner reaction is that she cannot escape from these torments, and she lives in perpetual fear that the therapist will finally abandon her. She seems transfixed in not being able to improve her lot, or to come to grips with her own reality, or to see herself as possessing any trait that another person could love or find happiness in. She is thus caught up in the vortex of a demeaning relationship with a therapist who offers her nothing but vituperation and a tentacular hold on her life, thus keeping her virtually imprisoned.

What is it that binds the woman to such a harrowing relationship? Why does it seem so impossible to break out of the bondage of the therapist? In part the answer has more to do with the woman's past than with the present. These are usually women who have been sexually abused during childhood by a sadistic father or stepfather or a divorced mother's current boyfriend or possibly some other close member of the family, such as an adolescent boy who is willing to take out his own sexual anger on a younger female child. In some cases the adolescent boy is emulating what he has already seen his father do to the young female child.

Typically the child attempts to communicate her plight to the mother, but also typically, the mother refuses to hear the problem and turns a deaf ear to any efforts the child makes to inform the mother of her fearful experiences. Not uncommonly, one finds that the woman patient has earlier in the therapy described for the treater the terrifying conditions that existed in her home where some male person in the family—usually father—was engaging in sexual abuse of the child and arousing in her a lasting fear of contact with men, not only sexually, but in what one would consider ordinary social interactions. One would expect the therapist to develop some empathic reaction, but with the abusing therapist, precisely the opposite happens. He instead uses the information to carry out with the patient the very interaction she has described as so painful and frightening.

What develops in the child is an obsessional disorder arising from the conviction that the horrible and frightening contact with the abusing figure in the family will continue forever, that there is no escape and no place to hide. There is only an inner despair born of her fears that each new occasion of assault will be worse than the one before. Not uncommonly, a child caught up in such troublesome sexual contacts will suffer regularly from nightmares or disturbing waking fantasies that shatter the child's equilibrium, leaving her feeling that she has no protection and that she must endure the hurtful abuse from within her own family. Such children often become morose, tearful, cautious, unwilling to talk with others because they believe their guilty secret, if discovered, will cause them more pain and fear. So a certain part of the child's psyche remains regressed, and while the patient grows older, she does not escape the memories or the fears of her troubled past.

THE REPETITION COMPULSION

It is not surprising, then, to discover that when women with such backgrounds later seek help from a therapist, and this therapist in turn uses his information to create for the patient another living nightmare in his efforts to gain sexual control, the patient is likely to develop disturbing regressive reactions. Typically such patients find themselves caught up in a web they had hoped to escape, and discovering that they are reliving the horrors of childhood, they sink into a depressive state that paralyzes their capacity to take action on their own behalf. It is as if the power that was held by the father (or other family member) has been transferred to the therapist, and the patient slips back into the old patterns of becoming fearful, reexperiencing the sources of one's own badness, and despairing of any significant change in one's fate. The patient then loses whatever control she had over her life, gives up on herself, and pliantly accepts whatever control the therapist places over her.

The reliving of past experiences that usually occurs following the sexualization of the treatment hours with the therapist brings about a fusion of past experiences with whatever is happening currently. At times the patient who is caught in this situation becomes confused about time or begins to see the therapist as if he were the father or whoever it was who introduced her to sexual contact. The patient may become that child again in the presence of the therapist, but her experience is peculiarly fused with the past, leading to uncertainty and confusion about what is past and what is present. This blurring of the patient's reality may persist for a period of time. In some cases patients have reported living in a kind of mesmerized state as if what happened in the patients' past childhood seduction is seen or felt as an ongoing process—a living out again of the fearful contact with the father or with some other agent responsible for the troubled condition of the child-self. Once the past has been resurrected in this way, it continues to return, sometimes weakly, but more commonly with the full force of the previous trauma, which then becomes fused with whatever troubled condition the sexualizing therapist brings to bear on the patient.

For some patients the situation is worse because they suffer from an invalidating depressive state that does not lift. Furthermore, such a depressive state may threaten a disintegration of the superego, and it is from this fear that the patient seems to be so anxiety-ridden. Not surprisingly, one sees a good deal of hatred in women who have been sexually abused, and they often come to treatment feeling empty and self-destructive. Searles (1979) and others have indicated that one reason therapists become caught up in a sexual approach to the patient is because they sense they cannot reach the core of the patient's problem and therefore fall into an acting out of their own problems: If they cannot reach the patient through their therapeutic skills, they will attempt to penetrate her in a different fashion. But again, such an approach must be based on some pathological narcissism on the part of the therapists that they would be so willing to give up their therapeutic technique and understandings and to replace them with a sadistically tinged sexual contact.

Furthermore, such activity by the therapist deepens the infantile depression such women usually suffer as a result of the early sexual abuse by the father. But it is also true that if the mother is depressed, the child may experience a loss, especially if the mother has been in good contact with the child earlier and the child was at that time able to develop a sense of power or at least well-being. But the mother's depression may reverse this process, the child may lose her own sense of integrity, may feel lost and abandoned by the mother whose depression the child now embraces. It is at this low point, when the child feels the loss of the mother as an inner trauma, that the child attempts to move toward an attachment to the father out of a longing for some kind of union.

It is the recapitulation of these circumstances in the therapeutic hour that the therapist may now exploit rather than analyze. The returning depression of the past, possibly spurred by current issues in the patient's life, gives the therapist an opportunity to become the loving substitute for mother by reawakening the patient's attachment to father. Generally speaking, such an approach to the patient only sets the patient back, most likely in the direction of the same depressive symptoms the patient suffered earlier in life. Indeed, it is this attachment to father, brought on by the mother's depressed and detached condition, that leads the patient to seek out a male therapist in the first place. It is as if the patient, in becoming overwhelmed by the infantile depression once again, now seeks out father to bring about a reparative reversal of the symptom.

But if the therapist introduces the "sexual solution" to the patient's problems, then one is likely to see in the patient a recapitulation of the child's earlier ego collapse when mother withdrew from the child. Experience indicates that such a disintegration is not likely to be easily overcome because the control issues in the patient's life are not attended to in any meaningful way. The introduction of sexual contact with the therapist leaves the patient helpless. As the patient begins to see the therapist as father, then the only means of maintaining integrity is to fall into a position of hatred—hating mother, hating father, hating the therapist, feeling as if one is surrounded by the hostility of others, all the while reliving with the therapist the trauma of the past.

The patient then withdraws into her own depressive anger and becomes literally unreachable. Here again Searles's notion that the therapist, having become frustrated by the patient's response to treatment, may introduce sexuality as a way of having some contact with the patient, is relevant, and this fact may offer an explanation of the loss of control. But one has to carefully consider that this form of sexual contact is usually made early in the treatment, so it is not so much that the therapist is using a means of last resort but that he more likely saw in the condition of the patient an easy mark for fulfilling his own sexual needs. Certainly the studies on sadomasochism reveal that if one agent assumes the role of the sadist, the other may be forced into the position of the masochist, and in the case of these women patients, the masochism has already been deeply implanted by a sexually abusing member of the family.

One is confronted in this situation with an unfortunate double bind in that the patient has no way of escaping from her frozen emotional condition, and the therapist seems to have no way to help the patient understand her own past. He seems capable only of acting out the past, a procedure that is neither therapeutic nor ultimately fulfilling for either patient or therapist. In fact, many of these women patients, because of the nature of their early experiences, have little capacity for love. If the patient's fixation is primarily on the mother—particularly the absent mother—then contacts with men, including father, are not likely to be satisfying. In certain instances, the patient is likely to reenact the sexual contact with father in the hour with the therapist, and at that point the therapist is confronted with a choice: He can either interpret for the patient what is going on or he can act it out. The point to be emphasized, however, is that this "recounting" of the past by the patient often results in the therapist's identification with the cruelty and the sadism of father or in some cases of mother. In the eyes of the patient, the therapist becomes the injurious parent, and in doing so opens the door to all the horrors and all the fears of the past.

It is this reenactment that triggers the patient's regressive feelings and results in a return of the past: the old fears, the sense of desperation, the inability to escape, the fragmentation of the psyche, the failed efforts to move away from these troublesome percepts, and the inner emptiness that leaves the patient feeling hopeless, especially because the child-woman patient has discovered that mother does not want to know what father is doing. It is this knowledge that so often keeps the patient from acting on her own behalf, and this issue in turn leads the patient back to her own childhood experiences with father's sexuality. The child's conviction, under such circumstances, is that no one is there for her and that the only protection she has is her ability to become numbed to the psychological pain she experiences.

This chapter has focused exclusively on the seduction of the female patient by the male therapist simply because much more is known about sexual boundary violations of this therapist-patient configuration than the others. The dynamics involved in female therapist–male patient dyads and those involving same-sex relationships must await further study.

Chapter 6

The Lovesick Therapist

Stuart W. Twemlow, M.D.
Glen O. Gabbard, M.D.

Harry Stack Sullivan (1954) felt that psychotherapy was the most difficult of all professional activities because it offered the patient a unique situation in which the therapist's own needs were excluded from the therapeutic arena. He felt that few individuals were suited for such work, and noted that

> ... there is no fun in psychiatry. If you try to get fun out of it, you pay a considerable price for your unjustifiable optimism. If you do not feel equal to the headaches that psychiatry induces, you are in the wrong business. It is work—work the like of which I do not know. (p. 10)

Every psychotherapist struggles with the temptation to seek personal gratification from the therapeutic situation. Buie (1982-83) observes that one of the central motivations for a career in psychotherapy is a wish to be relieved of one's sense of isolation and aloneness. Psychotherapists have a need for patients to provide them with a holding environment that sustains them. Buie notes that the psychotherapist "implicitly hopes that in meeting his patient's needs his own need for the kind of sustaining togetherness that mitigates depressive aloneness will be fulfilled" (p. 227). Untangling such motivations is one of the principal tasks of the therapist's own personal treatment experience.

While exploiting one's patient for sexual and emotional fulfillment is the most glaring example of deriving gratification from the psychotherapeutic relationship, less dramatic examples are far more common. From the time that Freud, perhaps unhappy in the healing role, suggested that psychoanalysis was a research tool as much as it was a treatment, a more ambiguous ethical concern has haunted the profession. Are therapists justified in making use of their patients for their own education, for case studies published in scientific papers, and for clinical material to be used in didactic seminars? Person (1983) reports on the reanalysis of two male patients who unexpectedly had each read about themselves in scientific papers that had been written by their first analysts. Although neither reacted negatively at the time of the discovery, in reanalysis each expressed the feeling that he had been "raped." The clinical purist might agree with Sullivan, who implies that the only gratifications a therapist may dutifully expect are the fee and improvement in the patient's symptomatic picture.

While we are not suggesting that using a patient for a case report or for one's own education is tantamount to exploitation, we are noting that a subtle continuum exists in the area of deriving personal gratification from one's patients. Psychotherapists are fond of regarding their unethical colleagues who engage in therapist-patient sex as "impaired," "sick," and, most of all, different. This continuum reminds us that the potential for exploitation of patients exists in all of us. It exists in activities that are generally considered professionally and ethically acceptable, and none of us can assume that he or she is immune to the temptation for exploitation.

Between us we have treated six offending therapists and 16 patients who have been abused by prior treaters. In addition, we have consulted on numerous other cases. It is our experience that many therapists who become involved in sexual boundary violations do not appear to suffer from disturbances that are sufficiently visible to have caused alarm in their colleagues.

Sexually abusing psychotherapists fall into three broad categories: the psychotic, the antisocial, and the lovesick. The psychotic group represents a very small subset of all offenders. A chilling case example conveys the gross disturbance typical of these cases. A clinical psychologist working on a girls' adolescent unit of a state mental hospital became convinced that God was speaking to him. He maintained that God had told him that his semen would confer eternal salvation on his patients, so he systematically set out to seduce every adolescent patient on his unit before finally being hospitalized himself.

The number of abusing therapists with antisocial features is considerably larger. These individuals are ruthless, are without remorse or empathy for their victims, and are the most frankly exploitative. Ethics committees have met with great frustration in attempting to rehabilitate these individuals, and many are ultimately forced to leave the profession.

Of the three groups, the lovesick (a broad category subsuming "normals," neurotics, and assorted personality disorders) are at once the most interesting and the most puzzling. How is it that reasonably well-functioning professionals become involved in a highly pathological and unethical relationship that can destroy their career and severely harm their patients under the guise of "true love"? In the Chapter 1 survey by Gartrell et al., 65 percent of the offenders stated that they had been in love with their patients, and 92 percent believed that the patients were in love with them. In a smaller study (Butler and Zelen 1977; Zelen 1985), 55 percent of a sample of 20 therapists who had been sexually involved with patients described a "total attraction, physically, emotionally, and intellectually." Both large surveys and detailed case studies (Holtzman 1984) portray a common scenario: A middle-aged male therapist, having difficulties with intimate relationships in his own life, falls in love with a female patient who is an average of 16.5 years younger (Holroyd and Brodsky 1977; Zelen 1985) and to whom he portrays himself as lonely, vulnerable, and needy. One can conservatively estimate that roughly one-half of the reported cases of therapist-patient sexual contact involve lovesickness.

LOVESICKNESS

While psychoanalytic writers have emphasized the pleasures of enduring commitment in the context of a mature genital relationship over the wild joys of passion, novelists, playwrights, and artists have thought otherwise. *Romeo and Juliet,* for example, might serve well as a literary model for this form of dyadic illness. However, this literary allusion immediately raises a vexing question: Are all cases of lovesickness pathological? Of course not. If they were, the overwhelming majority of the human population would have to acknowledge that they have suffered from this affliction at some point in their life. Before differentiating the pathological from the normal or healthy variety of lovesickness, we will first delineate the key characteristics of the lovesick state and discuss some of the underlying dynamics from a psychoanalytic perspective.

There has been extensive research on *limerence,* a term coined by Tennov (1979) in a research study of approximately 400 subjects who described the state of being in love. A psychoanalytic elaboration of this concept by Verhulst (1984) defines limerence as an "altered state of consciousness," characterized by an affect-dominated state of mind—in stark contrast with the ordinary language-dominated state. More accurately, this state often coexists with a language-dominated state of mind that is quite capable of structuring time sequentially and maintaining subject-object differentiation. Hence a lovesick individual may experience himself as fused with another individual and in an ecstatic, passionate state, on the one hand, while at the same time having the capacity to engage in language-dominated ego states, where such fusion would be unthinkable. As a reflection of this dual-state capacity, many a therapist has been known to conduct perfectly acceptable psychotherapy with other patients before and after he has sex with a patient in his office.

As we define it, lovesickness has the following basic phenomenological features.

Emotional dependence.   The need for each other is so great in lovesickness that each party will do virtually anything to be in the presence of his or her loved one. If one's lover cannot be physically present, one will pass the time by evoking an internal image of the missing party to assuage one's loneliness. In one such clinical instance, the patient would spend many hours dressing in front of a mirror, imagining how her therapist would reciprocate her feeling of love when he saw her. All reality becomes subservient to the intense emotional dependency. One patient commented, "I was drawn to him so much that we had a need to touch each other all the time." After a love relationship broke up between therapist and patient, the patient called her therapist, and through her tears of love and rage, shouted,

> I miss you terribly. It hurts so bad because it felt so good. I want to be back in your arms. My world seems empty without you. I want to see you and have you caress me and touch me and call me darling. It seems like it will never end (the pain of the loss). I pray for the day the memory will fade. I will be rid of you.

If this feeling of intense emotional dependency is reciprocated, the individual experiences happiness that approaches religious ecstasy. However, slight rejections lead to severe depression, suicidal ideation, and even suicide attempts. In one such situation, multiple suicide attempts were retrospectively related to very slight rejections by the therapist—for example, on one occasion the therapist did not greet his patient by her first name. It should be noted in passing that these lovesick states do not always involve sexual relationships. Frequently, intense performance anxiety may make sexual relations impossible. In other situations, the sexual contact may occur but is highly dysfunctional. For example, in a relationship where neither the patient nor the therapist had ever experienced a satisfactory sexual relationship, the sexual contacts in the therapist's office were always felt to be pressured by perfectionistic wishes and an intense fear that the specialness of the timeless moment would be lost. He had premature ejaculation while she faked an orgasm; but neither told the other of their lack of satisfaction.

Intrusive thinking. A couple stuck in the lovesick state often find that they can think of nothing but each other. Virtually every waking hour is occupied by intrusive thoughts. These frequently are fantasies with idealized or perfectionistic qualities reflecting a considerable denial of reality. One therapist was preoccupied with the visual image of his patient walking away from his office. He savored the memory of how her hips swayed from side to side, and he compared her to a "classic beauty," like a young Elizabeth Taylor. In reality, the patient was stocky, obese, and dowdy. This circumscribed suspension of reality testing may be why the state of being in love has often been compared to a psychosis.

Physical sensations. A variety of physical sensations may be present in the lovesick state. Commonly, one experiences a sensation of buoyancy, a feeling of "walking on air." A pounding pulse, dryness in the mouth, and tremulous hands or knees are also common. One therapist said he could feel his "heart in his throat" whenever his beloved entered his office. These physical sensations may also occur even in the absence of the partner when a mental image of him or her is brought to mind.

A sense of incompleteness. This feature is closely linked to the emotional dependence alluded to above. The individual often feels that he is not a whole human being without the other member of the dyad. The partner is idealized in such a way that all negative characteristics are regarded as positive. The perversity of it is typified in Emily Brontë's *Wuthering Heights,* where Katherine says about Heathcliff: "He is more myself than I am. Whatever our souls are made of, his and mine are the same." Almost all the lovesick patients and therapists that we have seen in treatment or consultation have experienced a sense that the missing partner completes some fundamental part of the personality. The descriptions are reminiscent of Aristophanes's account of the birth of love in the Symposium. Primordial man, according to this legend, was split in two as punishment for daring to defy the gods. The diminished creatures longed so desperately for their other halves that the gods took pity on them and granted them organs of generation through which they could, for brief moments, come together as one again and achieve wholeness. This sense of fusion with the partner is a phenomenological feature that lends itself to psychoanalytic understanding, as we will elaborate later.

Social proscription.   This feature may or may not be present in "normal" states of lovesickness, but it certainly characterizes all therapist-patient sexual relations. As portrayed so movingly in *Romeo and Juliet,* social proscription intensifies the excitement and dedication of the partners to each other. Risk-taking behavior further heightens the excitement. Juliet is baffled by the fact that "her only love is born of her only hate," as she tells her nurse. Romeo feels that the situation is so contradictory that it cannot be understood. The intensity of their love is highlighted by the quarreling between the two families, leading to their tragic and untimely deaths, which themselves were products of their fear that without one another they could not survive.

Many therapists and patients involved with each other have later commented that the very unavailability of one another under the circumstances intensified their longings. As one therapist put it, "The fact that a romantic relationship between us was ethically impossible filled me with a heartbreaking and sorrowful yearning." In Marshall Brickman's appropriately named 1983 film, *Lovesick,* Dudley Moore plays a middle-aged analyst who is immediately smitten by his beautiful young patient (Elizabeth McGovern). Despite the fact that he knows his patient is off limits, the analyst falls madly in love with her and seeks out his former analyst (John Huston) to get some fatherly advice. When his mentor suggests that he is experiencing counter-transference, the Dudley Moore character asserts that on the contrary, he is having "real feelings," as though there were some clear way of differentiating the two. In *Lovesick,* all the senior members of the analytic society who advise Moore to stop his love affair with McGovern are portrayed as buffoons who adhere to an antiquated and repressive code of ethics, and the audience applauds Moore's decision to defy the professional and ethical proscriptions of organized psychoanalysis and stroll off into the moonlight with McGovern at the end of the film (Gabbard and Gabbard 1987). Dudley Moore's character is portrayed as a hero who is sacrificing success and the trappings of his profession for "true love." Similarly, in real life the therapist and patient may feel that they have something so special that it transcends ordinary ethical and professional proscriptions. Like Dudley Moore in *Lovesick,* the therapist is likely to regard his profession's ethical code with contempt, viewing it as an unjust and unduly repressive attempt to stifle emotional spontaneity between patient and therapist.

Altered state of consciousness. As all of the foregoing features suggest, the lovesick state is not the therapist's ordinary state of consciousness. One abusing therapist described himself as "drugged or dreamlike when with the patient." This state-bound quality to lovesickness may partially explain the extraordinary risks that therapists often take. Therapists who are otherwise sober and careful individuals will suspend their ordinarily intact ego functions, such as judgment, while they are in this altered state of consciousness. It seems as though the romantic passion of the state sweeps away recognition of the substantial risks of the relationship.

A Psychoanalytic Understanding of Pathological Lovesickness

In some cases the therapist, particularly if antisocial features are present, may use the "true love" argument as a conscious rationalization for his behavior or as a feeble attempt to defend his position against ethical charges (Pope and Bouhoutsos 1986). The dynamics of these therapists can be linked to superego defects (Marmor 1976). However, many therapists genuinely believe that they are hopelessly in love with their patients. These therapists do not have lifelong histories of impulse-ridden behavior and chaotic disruptions of relationships such as those characteristic of antisocial personality disorder. For this group—the lovesick therapists—a more complex understanding is required.

Most psychodynamic formulations of the therapist involved in therapist-patient sexual relations derive from the Oedipus complex. Saul (1962) proposes that the contact is a form of benevolent parenting, an unconscious response to the patient's eroticized wish for a parent. Marmor (1976) postulates a reaction formation against inner feelings of masculine inadequacy and pseudohomosexual fears. Kardener (1974), one of the early researchers of the incidence of this problem, notes that estimates of incest in the general population— some 5–15 percent—are rather similar to his survey figures. The parallel nature of these figures lends itself to theorizing that therapist-patient sex is a direct acting out of an incestuous oedipal wish to have a forbidden lover.

Certainly the analogy to incest is appropriate. However, in our view the focus on oedipal dynamics does not do justice to the complexity of the clinical picture of lovesickness. For one thing, the symptomatology deriving from oedipal conflicts is heavily tinged with guilt, an affect that is remarkably absent in the lovesick therapist. The hallmark of the Oedipus complex is ambivalent, triangular object relations, characterized by jealousy, rivalry, and the capacity for whole-object relatedness. In the state of lovesickness, on the other hand, object ties are intensely dyadic rather than triangular. Moreover, whereas ambivalent oedipal relations are fused with negative feelings, the object relations of lovesickness are so idealized that they are completely free from contamination by any negative feelings whatsoever. "Badness" in oneself and in one's lover is denied, so neurotic guilt is absent. In the lovesick state, no one exists outside the intense passionate dyad, so rivalry is peripheral or absent. Finally, all the foregoing relates to the fact that fully rounded, ambivalently held, whole-object relations are not present in pathological lovesickness. The relationship is a part-self-representation connected with a part-object-representation—only the idealized aspects of self and object exist.

While oedipal themes are undoubtedly present in the lovesick therapist, our work with both therapists and patients who have been involved in therapist-patient sexual relations has convinced us that more primitive, preoedipal issues are of equal importance.

Love feeding. There are two traditions in the history of the psychoanalytic theory of technique. The oldest tradition, the one with which Freud is usually connected, asserts that cure occurs as a result of verbal explanations made by the analyst to the patient. The other tradition, typified by the British school of object relations, views the primary mechanism of cure as the internalization of a relationship (i.e., in the course of treatment the patient internalizes the therapist as a new internal object, one that modifies the patient's self- and object-representations). One erroneous extension of this latter tradition is the view that the therapist's task is to provide for the patient the love that the patient did not receive from her parents. Franz Alexander's (Alexander and French 1946) corrective emotional experience was designed to accomplish this task. Sandor Ferenczi promoted his Active Technique as "that of an affectionate mother" (Grubrich-Simitis 1986) who "gives up all consideration of one's own convenience, and indulges the patient's wishes and impulses as far as in any way possible" (p. 272). This assumption that the patient needs love may take the primitive form of actually sitting the patient on one's lap and feeding the patient as described by Sechehaye (1951).

Many therapists who become sexually involved with their patients do not experience guilt because they are convinced that they are providing their patient with a better parenting experience that will heal the pain and torment at the core of the patient's psyche. The idea that "the patient lacks love and I will feed her" involves a primitive concretization of several complicated metapsychological constructs. At the most primitive level it may take the form of the clinical psychologist mentioned above who felt that his semen would confer eternal salvation on the adolescent patients he was treating. Even at a more advanced level, the idea that the love of the therapist can cure the patient is alarmingly naive. Searles (1979) believes that many cases of therapist-patient sex derive from the patient's thwarting of the therapist's omnipotent strivings to heal the patient. When the therapist feels that his loving and caring help is not curative, he may resort to sexual relations as a despairing final effort.

Helping professionals frequently feel that they did not receive the love they deserved as children (Gabbard and Menninger 1988; Vaillant et al. 1972), and they may give to others what they feel they did not receive as children. As Buie (1982-83) suggests, this altruistic defense may mask an underlying wish to be loved and nurtured by one's patients. Grubrich-Simitis (1986) notes that Ferenczi was the son of a harsh mother and was perhaps trying to give the experience of an affectionate mother to his patients—an experience he did not receive as a child.

Hence the therapist who falls in love with his patient under the guise of "feeding" her with the love she missed may simply be gratifying his own long-denied yearnings for love. In this regard it is striking how often there is role reversal in the romantic relations of therapist and patient. In one such case, the therapist would often lie with his head in the patient's lap, speaking of his anxieties and troubles, even calling her his therapist. The patient was too terrified of rejection to act, but at times she had a powerful fantasy of throwing him off her.

Narcissus in the mirror.   It is often said that those who enter the field of psychotherapy have a narcissistic disturbance (Finell 1985; Miller 1981). Narcissistic problems may be overlooked in the therapist's personal analysis or therapy, and the practice of psychotherapy itself provides a number of narcissistic gratifications. The therapist who needs to be loved and idealized can always find patients who will fulfill that need. Claman (1987) feels that a narcissistic disturbance is at the root of many sexually abusing therapists. We share this view, one also supported by Smith's observations in Chapter 5. In fact, many of the so-called "normal" therapists who fall in love with patients and surprise their colleagues with their unethical behavior have probably been well-functioning narcissists who become lovesick over a patient in the midst of a life crisis. Many a therapist may enter the field because of a longing for selfobjects who will mirror him and sustain the therapist's self in a cohesive state.

Kohut (1971) used mirroring to refer to a developmental stage where the child's grandiose self-display is designed to capture the gleam in his mother's eye, by which Kohut meant an empathic and admiring response. In the classical myth of Narcissus, however, a different kind of mirroring is involved. Narcissus peers into the pool and falls in love with a reflection of himself. This usage of mirroring is also applicable to the lovesick therapist and his beloved patient. So-called "love at first sight" may reflect such a narcissistic experience where one feels that he sees himself in another person. Although not an instance of heterosexual romantic love, a well-described historical example of this phenomenon is the relationship between Bertrand Russell and Joseph Conrad (Hamilton 1979). Although the men were extraordinarily different politically, personally, and intellectually, they were instantly infatuated with each other when they met. While they actually were in the presence of each other very few times in the course of their lives, they always had the experience of a deep understanding when they gazed into each other's eyes. Hamilton speculates that this was related to a shared early parental loss at very similar age. He relates it to the concept of the doppelgänger or mystical double (Gabbard and Twemlow 1984). Each saw in the other a damaged self-representation that established a mutual reverberating sympathy.

This same instant rapport and connection may be involved in some cases of therapists who fall in love with patients. There is an unconscious perception that each member of the dyad can satisfy a need or ameliorate a conflict in the other. In one clinical example that came to our attention, when the therapist and patient stopped their sexual involvement, the patient was profoundly hurt and commented, "It's like a reenactment of my father's death." Her mother had been extremely sadistic and unsupportive, and her father had died at a time when the patient was very young so that she did not have her father as a buffer between a cannibalistic and symbiotic mother and the demands of external reality. The therapist had also lost his father at an early age, and although his mother had not been sadistic, she was inadequate and withdrawn so that he had similarly suffered a terrible loss following his father's death. In this therapist-patient dyad, the therapist supplied an idealized representation of the dead father and often actually intervened between the patient and her mother to prevent the latter's destructive and sadistic attacks. The patient supplied the therapist with a more emotionally spontaneous mother and a more responsive sexual partner (his wife was frigid).

Although in the foregoing example there was a striking similarity in the backgrounds of therapist and patient, such historical coincidences are not necessary for this narcissistic mechanism often found in lovesickness. Via projective identification, the therapist may project aspects of himself into the patient, who may then respond as though she actually is the projected self-representation. As described by Ogden (1979) this process occurs in three steps: (1) the projector projects a self- or object-representation into the recipient; (2) the recipient unconsciously identifies with the projected self- or object-representation and begins to behave accordingly as a result of interpersonal pressure exerted by the projector; and (3) the projector reintrojects the projected self- or object-representation after it has been psychologically processed and modified by the recipient of the projection. Kernberg (1987) adds that projective identification also has an element of control in which the projector attempts to control the recipient of the projection in a continuing effort to defend against intolerable experience.

A fictional account of this projective identification mechanism is described in Allen Wheelis's *The Doctor of Desire* (1987). In this provocative novel, Dr. Melville falls madly in love with a musician who comes to him for psychoanalysis. As he suffers endlessly in his lovesick state, he finally realizes the origins of his countertransference love in a blinding flash: "She is no other, she is I. In loving her I love myself, in rescuing her I redeem a part of myself—weak, frightened, feminine—of which otherwise I must be ashamed. . . . I have found an idealized portrait of my hidden self. . . . My lovelorn enslavement is to a lurking image in a dark mirror" (p. 112).

This tendency for the therapist to fall in love with his own projected reflection is intimately linked to a desire for union with some hidden, split-off aspect of oneself. The yearning for a patient may carry an unconscious meaning of a yearning for wholeness, with the belief that the patient, through the act of genital union, can provide that feeling of wholeness. Hamilton (1986) points out that projective identification is too often linked exclusively with bad and unacceptable aspects of oneself. Idealized aspects of the self may also be projected, resulting in a grandiose image of the recipient of the projection. When the therapist projects this idealized self-representation into the patient, an unspoken agreement transpires between therapist and patient:

> I like you to the extent that you are like I want you to be, and like I want to be myself. Provided we do not allow mundane external reality to intervene and spoil what we have, we can actually achieve a state of perfection as long as we maintain this special and unique relationship. What we have between us cannot be put into words, but we each know that when we are together, we experience a unique sense of wholeness.

This form of attachment is reminiscent of Freud's (1914) early description of narcissistic object choice, in which the patient's infantile self is projected onto the object and there is a blurring of the functions of self and object.

Ego boundary disturbance. As implied by the therapist's perception of aspects of himself in his patient and the feeling that he is incomplete without her, an ego boundary disturbance is part of the

lovesick state. Much of our understanding of ego boundary disturbances derives from the ego psychological formulations of Paul
Federn (1952). In his view, ego boundaries delineate what is "me"
from what is "not me." Federn conceptualized the ego boundary as a
peripheral sense organ, involving both mental boundaries and body
boundaries, that also discriminates that which is real from that which
is not real. Federn viewed the ego boundaries as flexible and perme-
able under certain conditions. Although less systematic in his understanding of boundary diffusion phenomena, Freud himself acknowledged this phenomenon in *Civilization and Its Discontents*: "There
are cases in which parts of a person's own body, even portions of his
own mental life—his perceptions, thoughts and feelings—appear
alien to him and as not belonging to his ego; there are other cases in
which he ascribes to the external world things that clearly originate in
his own ego and that ought to be acknowledged by it" (1930, p. 66).

The lovesick state, then, can be understood as a regression to a
pleasant boundary-less state that precedes the development of ego
boundaries. This primitive state prior to the elaboration of ego boundaries was referred to as the "medial ego feeling" by Federn. He felt
that this formed the nexus for the development of a general affect-
laden feeling tone, which he referred to as "buoyancy" (Rinsley
1962). The regression to this state may account for the therapist's
feeling of buoyant lightness or the experience that he is "walking on
air."

This disturbance in the ego boundary helps to explain the
"nonpsychotic loss of reality testing" that seems to take place in the
lovesick therapist. Accompanying the fusion with the patient is a lack
of ability to discriminate what is real from what is not real because of
the dysfunctional state of the ego boundary. This disturbance appears
to be state-bound and transient since the therapist is otherwise
nonpsychotic and is able to exercise good reality testing when his
beloved leaves his office and the next patient enters.

PERVERSION AND LOVESICKNESS

Much of the dynamics heretofore described apply equally to "normal" lovesickness, for example, the passionate crushes of adolescence. What differentiates the normal variety from the highly pathological form of therapist-patient sexual passion? The lovesick
therapist is not merely breaking an ethical code of his profession. He
is acting with extraordinary destructiveness to a person who has

placed her trust in him. He is ignoring the treatment of the symptoms that brought the patient to him, and he is seriously damaging (perhaps irreparably) her capacity to trust future treaters (not to mention destroying his own career). Studies now provide convincing evidence that at least 90 percent of patients who are victimized by therapists have serious residual harm (Bouhoutsos et al. 1983). In our experience, even suicide is a disconcertingly common outcome of therapist-patient sexual relations.

The key factor that differentiates normal lovesickness from therapist lovesickness is the perverse element in the latter. As Stoller (1985) defines perversion, an activity is perverse

> ... *if the erotic excitement depends upon one's feeling that one is sinning.* ... And, what exactly, is the sin? It is the same as for all sins: the desire to hurt, harm, be cruel to, degrade, *humiliate* someone (including, at levels of lesser awareness, the desire to harm oneself). (p. 7)

Stoller further notes that an act of risk taking creates the greatest excitement in the perverse individual. Finally, he classifies an activity as perverse if it does not lead to sustained intimacy.

By Stoller's definition, the activity of the lovesick therapist clearly qualifies as perversion. Feeling that he is sinning and taking an extraordinary risk heightens the excitement for the therapist. Even though the wish to harm and humiliate may be repressed, split off, or disavowed, there is always some measure of observing ego present that knows the relationship is incestuous at its core. Why else would there be such an awareness of sin or wrongdoing? Finally, the vast majority of relationships between therapists and patients do not, of course, end in lasting intimacy. Even those rare instances which result in marriage may ultimately end chaotically. In one instance that came to our knowledge, the patient sued the therapist after 10 years of marriage.

Stoller's definition does not depend as much on the overt behavioral aspects of the sex act as it does on the intent and the intrapsychic life of the perpetrator. A wide variety of sexual activities occur between the lovesick therapist and his patient, ranging from the mundane to the bizarre. Regardless of the nature of the sexual behavior itself, the sadistic wish to destroy is the perverse core of the lovesick therapist's relationship with his patient. It is this key feature that allows for differentiation from normal varieties of lovesickness. We have made the same observations as Smith in Chapter 5 that professions of love and passion often cover a core of cruelty, hatred, and sadism.

The patient may be similarly defending against a good deal of hatred and destructiveness while she is involved with the therapist. Many patients who have come to therapy for a second try after their traumatizing experience will acknowledge frankly and openly that these feelings lay just beneath the surface. Searles (1979) shares our view and connects therapist-patient sex with murderous urges in both patient and therapist toward one another. He believes that therapists frequently resort to sexual relations out of rage at the patient's confrontation of the therapist's unconscious omnipotent wish to heal. One woman, for example, defeated all of her male therapist's efforts to help her. She insisted that the only way he could possibly be of help was to bring her to orgasm through intercourse. She threatened suicide if he did not comply with her request. After considerable torment, the therapist eventually acceded to her request, only to fail to bring the patient to orgasm. She later involved a subsequent therapist in a similar enactment.

PREVENTION

Prevention of lovesickness in therapists and the countertransference acting out that accompanies it is a formidable task. Clearly, a personal treatment experience for the therapist is not a fool-proof method of prevention. The Chapter 1 survey by Gartrell et al. found that offenders were more likely than nonoffenders to have undergone therapy or analysis. Profiles of susceptible therapists, such as those by Brodsky in Chapter 2 and by Pope and Bouhoutsos (1986), provide some guidelines for detecting which therapists might be at risk. The middle-aged male therapist, who is in the midst of a divorce or other problems in his intimate relationships should be alert to any tendencies toward overinvolvement with his patients. Does he inappropriately disclose aspects of his personal life to his patients? Does he think about a particular patient when she is not in the office with him? Does she enter his dreams? Does he begin to think that what his patient needs is love to make up for the lack of love she received in childhood? Finally, does he begin to think that he sees aspects of himself in his patients?

The primary difficulty with preventing therapist-patient sexual intimacy is that all of these questions must be asked by the therapist himself. Many of them are simply standard questions that every well-trained therapist uses to monitor his countertransference on a continual basis. However, the fact remains that no one can monitor these internal states other than the therapist himself. If the therapist does not seek out help at the first sign of these warning signals, he will rapidly descend into the chasm of lovesickness and no longer be amenable to help. Moreover, we are aware of some therapists who developed lovesickness while they were in regular supervision and simply withheld the information about the developing sexual relationship from their supervisors. These therapists felt that the relationship was so special that no supervisor could truly understand it. They concealed the information from supervision precisely because they did not want to stop the sexual relationship.

One prophylactic measure—one that therapists must enforce for themselves—is the avoidance of nonsexual dual roles with patients. A therapist-patient relationship should be a strictly professional one that is not contaminated with financial deals (other than fee arrangements) or various forms of socializing outside the therapy hour. An extensive questionnaire survey of 4,800 psychiatrists, psychologists, and social workers (Borys and Pope, in press) revealed that therapists involved in nonsexual boundary violations during psychotherapy are at an increased risk of becoming sexually involved with their patients.

While education about ethical problems in the practice of psychotherapy is important, if not essential, in training programs and continuing education workshops, the surveys reported in this book indicate that inadequate training is not the main problem. The narcissistic disturbance in the lovesick therapist is so pervasive among psychotherapists in general (see Buie 1982-83; Finell 1985; Miller 1981) that we would be hard pressed to delineate some point on the continuum at which a therapist's wish to receive certain affirming responses from his patient becomes so extreme that it places him at risk for falling in love with the patient and acting out his sexual wishes with her. Psychotherapists would do far better to assume that everyone is at risk and to engage in a continual intrapsychic monitoring process as part of their professional practice.

The data in Chapter 1 by Gartrell et al. indicate that only 41 percent of offenders sought out consultation because of their sexual involvement. Obviously, we have no data on the number of therapists who seek out consultation before getting involved as a way of preventing it. The therapist who wishes to seek help may be faced with a dilemma. As Pope (1987) points out, neither consultation nor supervision provide the extensive privilege under some state laws that the therapist-patient relationship provides. The therapist may wish to enter psychotherapy rather than pay for supervision or consultation simply to assure himself that whatever he says will be held in strict confidence. This situation may change in the near future, however, as many states are currently considering whether to allow either mandatory or discretionary reporting of therapist-patient sex even when therapist-patient privilege applies, similar to the current situation in most states regarding child abuse. For those who do seek out therapy, Pope (1987) has provided a useful model of intervention.

Finally, nothing can be more important than attention to one's private life. Far too many therapists put more energy into treatment relationships than into their marriages, where one can rightfully expect to seek personal gratification. The best prophylaxis is a satisfying personal life.

Chapter 7

Individual Psychotherapy for Victims of Therapist-Patient Sexual Intimacy

Kenneth S. Pope, Ph.D.
Glen O. Gabbard, M.D.

This chapter on individual psychotherapy with patients who have been sexually intimate with a prior therapist supplements Chapter 4, which addressed the evaluation of such patients. It draws from other published guides to individual treatment (Pope and Bouhoutsos 1986), but it also extends them.

The damage caused by sexual contact with the therapist can be so complex and pervasive, the needs of the individual patient so personal and idiosyncratic, and the vicissitudes of psychotherapy so difficult to pin down, that there can be no "by the numbers" guide. However, this chapter attempts to highlight a few of the major issues that any therapist working with victims of sexual exploitation by a previous therapist must face.

COMPETENCE

Psychotherapeutic work with these patients requires specialized knowledge, training, and experience. Numerous pitfalls await the inexperienced or inadequately trained therapist at every turn. When these pitfalls are not avoided, the subsequent therapy can not only fail to help the victim, but can also "re-victimize" and further damage the patient. As a bare minimum, clinicians who assume these treatment responsibilities need to be thoroughly familiar with the current theory, research, and treatment techniques, and to consult with therapists experienced in this area. Clinicians without specialized education, training, and experience should no more attempt unsupervised work in this area than they would, without adequate preparation and support, attempt biofeedback therapy with hypertensive patients, psychoanalytically oriented play therapy with young children, or outpatient psychotherapy with elderly patients at high risk for suicide. Unfortunately, we are familiar with a number of instances in which a patient has been seriously revictimized by subsequent therapists who were unfamiliar with this area of practice.

Openness, Honesty, and Clarity of Communication

One of the most fundamental prerequisites for effective therapy with these patients is the subsequent therapist's clarity and honesty of communication. The patient's relationship with the exploitative therapist involves serious boundary violations, muddled tasks, and confused communications. As one patient remarked, "It was as if everything took place in the dark. I wasn't sure who I was or where I was. I didn't understand what he was doing. I didn't know what was going on." The subsequent therapy must take place in a "well-lit room." Everything must be open and aboveboard.

Moreover, the patient's relationship with the prior therapist involved a devastating violation of trust. The subsequent therapist must be a stable and trustworthy figure. Therapists who are in the midst of a personal life crisis, and who therefore may be unusually vulnerable or needy, might do well to refer such patients elsewhere. The first task of the therapist must be to create a "holding environment" (Winnicott 1965) in which trust can gradually develop. As a result of their experiences with exploitative therapists, patients will often be extremely suspicious of any subsequent therapist, no matter how exemplary his or her reputation may be. Accusations that the therapist is "holding back," or is "just saying something because the books say you have to say that," or is "setting me up, just like my last therapist" are frequent. An approach of rigorous clarity and honesty—even if it appears to be repeatedly and vigorously rejected by the patient—is essential in helping the patient to heal from the prior abuse.

Therapists must ensure that they are truly prepared to listen carefully to the patient. As Pope and Bouhoutsos (1986) note:

Hearing complaints about a colleague is likely to elicit uncomfortable feelings of shock, anxiety, dismay, or disbelief. Such feelings may lead a subsequent therapist to screen out further information. The patient may discern, on the basis of the therapist's questions, comments, facial expressions, or body language, that this topic is taboo. The phenomenon is similar to that of some parents who are reluctant to listen to their children reveal that a kindly uncle has made sexual advances. It is also similar to the dynamics that make some therapists seemingly insensitive to their patients' tacit messages of suicidal intent. Therapists must convey their openness and attentiveness to anything the patient has to say. (p. 82)

The subsequent therapist must ensure that no subject is taboo, that anything the patient has to talk about is genuinely heard.

Finally, listening implies an open-minded receptivity to the unique aspects of the patient's experience. If the therapist assumes a priori that he or she knows how the patient experienced the sexual relationship with a previous therapist, such an assumption probably will lead to technical errors and an inability to empathize with the patient's experience. Therapist-patient sexual contact is a highly complex phenomenon that produces different reactions in different patients. In one instance, for example, the therapist offered the following observation to the patient, "You must have felt angry and exploited by Dr. _____." The patient looked puzzled and responded, "On the contrary, it was the most comforting relationship I've ever had." The therapist's attempt to empathize with the patient's experience turned out to be nothing more than an imposition of his preconceived notions onto the patient's experience.

GENDER

A frequent focus of the patient's concern during the initial contacts with the new therapist is the therapist's gender. This issue needs to be openly discussed before an agreement is made to work together. It is important to stress to the patient that there is no particular gender pairing that, in and of itself, seems to invariably promote or to preclude effective therapy with victims of prior abuse. Some patients, for example, may feel it is impossible to work with a subsequent therapist who is of the same gender as the offending therapist. Others may feel that working with a subsequent therapist who is of the same gender as the offending therapist will help them to work through the trauma more effectively and thoroughly.

Whatever the patient's feelings about this issue, they should be viewed as important and should be discussed openly. Furthermore, ultimately it is the patient who should and must make the decision about whether he or she does or does not want to work with a subsequent therapist of the same or opposite gender.

CHILDREN AS PATIENTS

Although virtually all of the published work concerning the treatment of victims of therapist-patient sexual intimacies focuses exclusively on adult patients, the needs of minor patients should not be overlooked. A national study by Bajt and Pope (1988) found that a substantial amount of sexual exploitation by therapists involved patients who were minors. Slightly more (56 percent) of these children were female, with a mean age of 13 years, ranging between 3 and 17 years. The male victims had an average age of 12 years, ranging from 7 to 16 years.

One important way in which subsequent treatment of minor patients differs is the legal context. As this chapter is written, therapist-patient sexual intimacy involving adults is a crime in only a handful of states. However, sexual involvement with minor patients is a crime in all 50 states. Moreover, the subsequent treating therapist may be legally required to report such sexual involvement to the legal authorities as child abuse. Such reports may vastly complicate the treatment. Second, the countertransference reactions of shock and disbelief, rescue fantasies, and other responses, which are discussed later in this chapter, may be much more pronounced. Third, the child's limited linguistic and other cognitive abilities, which are not fully developed and which draw upon a smaller basis of experience than the adult's, tend to make the trauma much more difficult to work through. The child was and remains exceptionally vulnerable.

In general, forms of play therapy (for younger children) and approaches specially developed for treatment of incest victims and other sexually abused children seem useful for minors who have been sexually intimate with a therapist.

CONFIDENTIALITY, PRIVILEGE, AND RECORDS

Even victimized patients who are absolutely certain that they would never file a formal complaint against their previous therapist may change their minds. It is critically important that patients understand clearly the degree to which filing a formal complaint, such as a malpractice suit or a letter to a licensing board, may waive their rights to confidentiality and privilege. Subsequent therapists must understand that anything they write in the chart may be subject to subpoena, may be read in open court, and may be extremely influential in the outcome of any court case or formal hearing. In some cases, in response to the understandable mistrust that patients have developed toward therapists, subsequent clinicians have found it useful and therapeutic to allow victimized patients to read over their charts. In some instances, it may be a useful practice to routinely show every note to the patient prior to filing it. Reading the notes in the presence of the therapist may help patients to feel that the therapist is "leveling" with them and not saying one thing to the patient and writing something different in the chart.

THE FOCUS OF TREATMENT

As suggested in Chapter 4, the first task of subsequent psychotherapists is a careful and comprehensive evaluation of the patient's condition. The treatment plan should be based on the results of this assessment and should have a clear focus. Patients who have been sexually exploited by a prior therapist may manifest multiple problems. The actual abuse may be a major presenting complaint of the patient or it may be regarded as a minor or peripheral issue at the beginning of treatment. The patient's primary concerns may revolve around the breakup of a marriage, symptoms of depression and/or anxiety, or loneliness. As a general rule, it is important to keep in mind that the more distressed, dysfunctional, or otherwise impaired the individual was prior to sexual involvement with the therapist, the more pervasive and lasting the damage produced by the sexual involvement tends to be.

   In terms of the expressive-supportive continuum, the psychotherapy should initially be of an ego-supportive nature. Regardless of the extent to which the patient identifies the sexual boundary violation as a major presenting problem, the patient's ego has nonetheless been overwhelmed by a traumatic experience. Attempts to be interpretive or exploratory early on may be perceived as attacks or intrusions that reactivate the trauma. In the opening and much of the middle phase of psychotherapy, the experiencing, and ultimately the internalizing, of a trusting, respectful, nonintrusive relationship is far more important than accurate explanatory interpretations. After a solid therapeutic alliance is formed, and this may take a very long time indeed, exploration of unconscious aspects of the situation may be useful.

Adjunctive Forms of Treatment

Many patients will respond better to individual therapy if it is augmented by concurrent group therapy. However, since this modality is considered in detail in Chapter 8, we will not discuss the use of group psychotherapy here except to say that it may be a valuable adjunct. Other useful resources to consider include mediation, self-help groups, and advocacy groups (see Pope and Bouhoutsos 1986). These adjunctive methods can help the patient feel less isolated, which in and of itself may have therapeutic benefit. Moreover, through contact with others, the patient comes to view the individual therapist as less of a "one-and-only lifeline." This broadening of the support network may make it easier for the patient to experience and manage feelings of dependency.

Discontinuations and Interruptions

It is not uncommon for these patients to quit therapy abruptly. While some may return from time to time to the same therapist, others may attempt to return to therapy repeatedly, each time with a new therapist. Unfortunately, every new therapy experience is doomed to failure because the patient is unable to sustain a therapeutic relationship due to insufficient anxiety tolerance, the reawakening of the trauma from the prior victimization, or simply the fact that the subsequent therapist is human rather than perfect. A subgroup of victims may never be able to resume psychotherapy.

It is crucial for subsequent therapists to avoid at all costs a critical attitude about the patient's inability to continue therapy. The therapist must rely on whatever interventions are most helpful in conveying an attitude that the door is always open for return. Responses based on the therapist's sense of possessiveness, abandonment, authoritative omniscience (e.g., "I know what's best for you, so you'd better stay in therapy with me"), wounded pride (e.g., "There must be something wrong with me as a therapist or else this patient wouldn't be leaving now"), or judgmental criticism are unlikely to be helpful.

GROUND RULES FOR THERAPIST-PATIENT INTERACTIONS

Patients may experience great difficulty feeling safe during the therapeutic sessions. Some may actively berate themselves for being so stupid and gullible as to let themselves be "set up" for abuse by yet a second therapist. Subsequent therapists can explore with their patients possible ground rules that might help them feel more safe, particularly during the earlier stages of therapy. Some patients, for example, respond well to a policy in which all physical contact is avoided. Such patients may be afraid that even the most innocuous and nonerotic contact, such as shaking hands, has sexual overtones or is a prelude to a sexual advance. Physical contact with the therapist may evoke vivid and terrifying flashbacks, intrusive thoughts, or unbidden images. Other patients may respond well to an explicit initial ground rule in which the therapist agrees not to ask any probing questions about the patient's sexual history, habits, desires, or fantasies. Part of this explicit ground rule is that the patient is at any time free to talk about sexual issues in any way that he or she sees fit—it is the therapist who agrees to refrain from raising the topic, from asking any leading questions, or from directing the focus of therapy in a way that the patient experiences as intrusive and dangerous.

FITTING THE PACE OF THERAPY TO THE PATIENT

Perhaps as an extension of the ground rules previously discussed, an exceptionally important principle is to allow patients to work at their own pace. There may be times when they are so overwhelmed by the cognitive and affective sequelae of their involvement with the prior therapist that it is all they can do to make it to a session. They may find themselves unable to talk at all, and may find it too overwhelming—even assaultive—for the therapist to fill the silence. Simply sitting in the presence of the therapist—and reassuring themselves that the therapist will not become sexual with them or otherwise behave in an assaultive manner—may help to calm their confusion and distress and to enable them to engage in more active exploration during later sessions.

On the other hand, some patients will experience silence as cold, critical, and rejecting. In the absence of verbalizations, the patient assumes the worst. Such patients may find periodic inquiries supportive rather than intrusive. They reassure such patients that the therapist has not in fact abandoned them. A reasonable practice is to ask the silent patient what he or she would find most helpful as a response to the prolonged silence.

AVOIDING THE DUAL ROLE OF THERAPIST-ATTORNEY

Too often therapists intentionally or unintentionally block or dissuade their patients from learning about and acting on their legal rights. Legislation may help to ensure that therapists carry out their responsibilities in this regard. Chapter 1448 of Section 728 of the California Business and Professions Code, for example, states:

> Any psychotherapist or employer of a psychotherapist who becomes aware through a patient that the patient had alleged sexual intercourse or alleged sexual contact with a previous psychotherapist during the course of a prior treatment, shall provide to the patient a brochure promulgated by the department which delineates the rights of, and remedies for, patients who have been involved sexually with their psychotherapist.

Whether or not to file a formal complaint with the civil courts, a licensing board, or an ethics committee is always and only the patient's decision. The dilemma of being in the dual role of the patient's therapist and the protector of one's profession is further addressed in Chapter 10.

EDUCATION

Some patients respond exceptionally well to a therapeutic approach that includes an educational component. As patients educate themselves about the phenomenon of therapist-patient sex, about its prevalence, consequences, and treatment, they often develop an increased sense of control. What has happened to them becomes less mysterious and therefore less overwhelming. For some patients, of course, this process is similar to the use of intellectualization as a defense. It may still prove to be a useful and adaptive defense during the early stages of therapy, however; and it may enable these patients to overcome their psychological pain and paralysis and to progress to still more effective methods of coping.

Furthermore, reading about the degree to which this phenomenon is prevalent and about the experiences of other patients who have been sexually exploited can help patients to overcome their persistent feelings of isolation. Our own experience suggests that first-person accounts may have the most profound and therapeutic impact and therefore may serve as the best initial readings. These books humanize and personalize the concepts that other works address in a more theoretical or research-oriented manner.

COGNITIVE DYSFUNCTION

The flashbacks, intrusive thoughts, unbidden images, nightmares, and other cognitive dysfunctions may be among the most pressing and difficult aspects of therapist-patient sex syndrome to treat. Some patients find that these phenomena intensify during the periods between sessions and create an almost complete inability to function in addition to intense distress. For some patients, these cognitions related to their prior therapy are so intense, terrifying, and persistent that they believe only suicide can interrupt the bombardment. Indeed, in our experience disabling anxiety verging on panic may be a significant warning to the therapist that a highly lethal suicide attempt is imminent.

Pope (1985) reports that many of these patients seem to find it helpful to devote about an hour each day to reviewing and recording these cognitions as part of the process of working through. Some find it better to use a tape recorder, while others prefer a notebook. The patients may then bring either the tapes or the notebook to therapy, if they wish, or simply discuss the content with their therapist. The potential advantages of this approach are:

1. It helps patients to take a more active role in the recovery process and a more active (and less helpless) stance vis-à-vis the negative mental images.
2. It enables patients to structure their time and activities.
3. It helps patients to direct and control these cognitions (and alter their reactions to them).
4. It helps patients to internalize the therapeutic process.
5. It helps patients to learn the therapeutic process of translating images into words, a significant step toward understanding and integration (Horowitz 1976, 1978; Meichenbaum 1978; Singer and Pope 1978).

More elaborate methods—involving cognitive-behavioral techniques, imagery therapies, and "reconstruction and review"—for ad-

dressing these aspects of cognitive dysfunction are presented by Pope
and Bouhoutsos (1986).

TRANSFERENCE AND COUNTERTRANSFERENCE
IN THE SUBSEQUENT THERAPY

The countertransference experiences of the subsequent therapist often present the most difficult obstacles to the effective treatment of
patients who have been exploited by previous therapists. These reactions are strikingly similar to those experienced by therapists who
treat victims of intrafamilial incest. Ganzarain and Buchele (1986,
1988), based on their extensive experience treating incest victims,
identify the following feelings as typical countertransference reactions: shock and disbelief, excited curiosity, erotic fantasies, guilt
related to those fantasies, a need to blame the perpetrator, and rescue
fantasies. In Sonne's discussion of countertransference in Chapter 9,
she notes that a desire to be a perfect therapist evoked by the victims
of therapist-patient sex may lead to a tendency on the therapist's part
to become overindulgent and to refuse to set limits.

Transference-countertransference in the psychotherapy of these
patients can best be understood as repetitions. As Smith describes in
Chapter 5, the women who are abused by therapists are often unconsciously recreating childhood experiences in which fathers or other
men exploited them similarly. When these women come to a subsequent therapist, the same unconscious reenactment is a potential to
which the therapist must be attuned. Via projective identification (see
Chapter 6), therapists may feel themselves becoming sexually
aroused by the patient or may find themselves saying or doing things
that they do not ordinarily do. In other words, the therapist may begin
to behave like an internal object of the patient that has been unconsciously projected into him or her as the therapy develops. These
reactions may be subtle and may be evoked by equally subtle
behaviors of the patient. For example, one therapist realized that he
was inching his chair closer to the patient in response to her tendency
to speak in a quiet voice with her head down during the sessions.

Erotic countertransference reactions are often—but not always—in response to the patient's erotic transference feelings for the
therapist. When the sexual feelings engendered by these patients
arise, they may create such discomfort in the therapist that a variety
of defensive maneuvers may be employed to deal with that discomfort. The therapist treating these patients must be open to such feel-

ings and regard them as having valuable diagnostic information like any other transference-countertransference paradigm in therapy. By remaining open to these feelings, the therapist may gain a glimpse of the patient's internal object relations and the ways in which the patient's inner world was involved in the prior sexual exploitation.

Moreover, if therapists cannot deal with their own sexual feelings, patients are likely to receive very little help in dealing with theirs. Patients may respond to the emergence of sexualized feelings toward the subsequent therapist with anxiety, shame, guilt, and terror. They may feel out of control and may fear that the new therapist, like the old, will exploit their vulnerabilities. When therapists begin to experience sexual attraction toward patients, they may feel guilty, anxious, or confused, and may find themselves acting in an unconsciously seductive or otherwise sexualized manner. On the other hand, they may feel so overwhelmed by anxiety about responding to the feelings that they withdraw from the patient and behave in a cold, detached manner. For example, when patients begin to recount experiences with the previous therapist, subsequent therapists may note ' a voyeuristic excitement that makes them uncomfortable and leads them to change the subject. Patients in such cases will rightly infer that the therapist could not handle the topic and so they may choose not to return for the next session. Other therapists deal with their erotic excitement by projecting all sexual feelings into the patient and viewing them as present in only one member of the dyad.

For any patient to experience an erotic transference is, of course, entirely normal and expectable in the course of psychotherapy. For a victimized patient to experience transference of feelings connected with a prior therapist to a subsequent therapist is also completely normal and expectable. Therapists must be sufficiently clear and responsible about their own reactions, about the nature and task of therapy, and about the normal reactions of patients who have been sexually victimized. They must communicate respect for and acceptance of any feeling a patient may have while maintaining a safe and supportive environment in which the patient is protected (and feels protected) against the exploitation of those feelings.

Faced with the complexity of the therapist-patient sexual phenomenon, another common countertransference reaction is a tendency to stereotype and simplify. As Ganzarain and Buchele (1986) note, "In an effort to avoid chaos, clinicians may artificially narrow their focus and, instead of realizing the multiple kaleidoscopic views of the complex problem of incest, may adopt stereotypes in an effort to understand it" (p. 562). Patients abused by therapists are likely to experience a wide range of feelings in the course of subsequent therapy. They may love and hate the therapist at the same time. They may feel abandoned by the therapist and yearn to return. They may experience murderous wishes toward the therapist. Clinicians must be open to all of these experiences as valid and expectable. Ganzarain and Buchele (1986) warn,

> If the countertransference reactions cause the therapist to be caught in a simplistic, categorizing view of what the patient's experience is, then what is omitted probably will be acted out. (p. 563)

By maintaining an open-minded view that does not stereotype or narrow the possibilities involved in the patient's reaction, the therapist may increase his or her discomfort, but at the same time the therapist's ability to accurately empathize with the patient's experience will be increased. It cannot be overstressed that the therapist who treats such patients will greatly benefit from having had a treatment experience of his or her own and by taking advantage of opportunities for consultation and supervision from therapists experienced in this kind of work.

Chapter 8

An Example of Group Therapy for Victims of Therapist-Client Sexual Intimacy

Janet L. Sonne, Ph.D.

In response to the troubling statistics reported in the earlier chapters in this volume, the Post-Therapy Support Project (PTSP) was established at the UCLA Psychology Clinic to provide group psychotherapy for people who had been involved sexually with their therapists. The rationale for group treatment of these clients was based on the premise that the exposure to other individuals who had had similar experiences might (1) reduce the person's sense of isolation and (2) invoke a sense of group objectivity that would be helpful in alleviating individual guilt and self-blame concerning the intimacy.

The PTSP groups consisted of respondents to newspaper articles, public announcements, and professional and personal referrals. Project staff interviewed all candidates and asked each potential group participant to complete a Minnesota Multiphasic Personality Inventory (MMPI). Project staff established specific criteria, discussed later in this chapter, that they considered to be contraindicative of group treatment. Then, after determining candidates' suitability, staff briefed clients on the nature of the group and invited those still interested to participate.

Project staff members included advanced graduate students in clinical psychology and licensed clinical psychologists. Students provided assessment and treatment services, and the psychologists served as therapists and as consultants. This chapter will outline and discuss many critical issues encountered by the UCLA project staff in the group psychotherapy with clients who had been sexually involved with their previous therapists.

GROUP TREATMENT FUNCTION

In general, group treatment may serve any of three functions. First, group psychotherapy can focus on the discovery and resolution of maladaptive individual and interactional dynamics. Second, therapy may aim to provide manifest psychosocial support and explicit education concerning a particular problem. And third, especially appropriate to the group treatment of concerns that raise ethical and legal dilemmas, therapy may provide clients with ethical/legal advocacy and even assistance with litigation preparation.

The group treatment of clients who have been sexually involved with their previous therapists legitimately may serve any one or combination of these functions. It is crucial for a number of reasons, however, that the treatment staff determine a priori the group function(s). First, clients need to be informed of the treatment emphasis before the treatment begins. Clearly, a focus on the emotional and psychological factors surrounding the sexual intimacy with a therapist demands a different involvement from clients than a focus on clients' ethical and legal rights and the avenues of recourse. Second, the treatment staff should have in mind the priority of the function of the group in order to avoid potential counterproductive conflicts while the treatment is in process. For instance, focus on the ethical and legal rights of clients likely will generate significant anger for some group members. While the anger may be appropriate and motivating for the pursuit of legal recourse by clients, the expression of anger by some may inhibit others who continue to feel quite protective of and loving toward their previous therapists. And third, the treatment staff needs to assess the potential detrimental effects for the client of its involvement in the litigation process, both in terms of the need for the "special overinvolvement" of the staff beyond the usual therapy setting (i.e., in court) and for the staff to produce treatment records to the court once subpoenaed.

The PTSP groups were primarily intended to provide support and education. When appropriate, the treatment did also address specific psychological dynamics. The staff, however, specifically avoided litigation advocacy or preparation in an effort to avoid potential conflict with the first two functions. Clients interested in or concerned with litigation were referred to appropriate resources.

GROUP TREATMENT PARAMETERS

Time-limited versus open-ended.   Psychotherapy groups may be either time-limited or open-ended and each has advantages and disadvantages. The time-limited group, by definition, meets regularly for several weeks and then terminates. The advantages of this group type with this specific clinical population is that the groups have a relatively stable membership and they are more highly structured in terms of the time commitment required of the participants. The clear disadvantage is that it may not be possible to address all of the issues that members are likely to bring to the meetings. On the other hand, the open-ended group continues to meet indefinitely until the group decides to disband. While allowing the group more latitude to define its own pace to address problems and, perhaps, more complete coverage of problems, the open-ended group must contend with inevitable member attrition over time, as well as the potential burnout of the staff and group participants working on the variety of complex issues.

For its first group, the UCLA project introduced a format that staff expected to provide a compromise between open-ended and time-limited. Group participants were asked to commit to meeting for 8 weeks (giving the group a clear time structure), at which time the group would decide whether to continue or not (allowing for the possibility of extended exploration). Unfortunately, the project established no specific guidelines with which to decide whether the group would continue or disband. Thus, at the 8th week, most members chose to terminate while a very few wished to continue. The project staff decided that there were too few who wanted to resume to work beneficially in a group process. The project staff decided then that following groups would be time-limited, meeting for 8 weeks.

Open versus closed.   Therapy groups also may be closed or open to new members as the group progresses over time. This parameter appears especially significant in the open-ended group format. The project staff anticipated the problems that the new clients would have in joining a cohesive group and determined that accessing new members would be highly disruptive to the ongoing group process. The project groups were closed.

Session frequency and length. These two parameters necessitated the project staff's consideration of the delicate balance of its response to the needs of this clientele versus the clients' hesitancy to trust and commit. Some members reported a desire for frequent meetings to help cope with their intense reactions to their experiences. However, others described feelings of dread and anxiety as the meeting time approached, feelings that were often difficult to cope with. The project groups met once weekly for 90 minutes, which appeared to provide an acceptable balance for the members.

Fees. Fee setting and collection presented the project staff with an unexpected countertransference issue. The group therapists and project staff began the group treatment with the implicit desire to provide better therapists than those who had exploited the clients, perhaps even perfect therapists. This desire appeared to contribute, at times, to the project staff's tendency to be overly accommodating to clients' wishes or demands. At the same time, several clients entered the group angry and disappointed, with the sense that they had previously wasted their time and money on therapy that had had a destructive influence. Some clients requested that they pay no fee or a very low fee for the group treatment regardless of their ability to pay. The project staff at first was tempted to waive or reduce fees but did return to clinic policy and adhere to the established sliding-scale fee structure based on ability to pay.

The Group Therapists

Number of therapists and therapists' sex and professional status. The staff carefully considered several issues regarding the therapists who were to conduct the group treatment. Because the vast majority of the clients were females who had been exploited by male therapists (though there were exceptions), the staff decided that female therapists may evoke less initial resistance than male therapists with this already sensitive client population. Cotherapists led the groups, primarily in anticipation of the complexity and intensity of the group process. Each therapist represented a different training level: (1) advanced graduate training in clinical psychology and (2) licensed psychologist. Although not anticipated by the staff, this arrangement allowed for easier joining of the group members with the therapists. As an expression of their understandable initial mistrust, some clients challenged the therapists' level of competency and motivation for leading the group. A licensed psychologist was perceived by some as more competent and less likely to be "in this for the training hours." On the other hand, some group members expressed discomfort with the perceived power of licensed therapists and clearly related more easily to the graduate student therapist.

Therapists' activity levels. The group therapists tended to be active from the beginning of the first group, an orientation that proved to be quite advantageous both as treatment progressed and in subsequent groups. Again, primarily in response to clients' substantial mistrust of the therapists and the therapy process, project therapists interacted in ways that promoted clarity regarding their roles, motivations, and actions. Although the therapists were self-disclosing, they remained vigilant for the kind of inappropriate self-disclosure that would likely cause role blurring between therapist and client, role blurring similar to that which occurred in the sexually intimate therapy. The distinction between appropriate and inappropriate therapist self-disclosure was determined theoretically by whether the disclosure would promote the clients' sense of understanding of the therapeutic interaction or merely enhance the therapist's sense of well-being. For instance, the therapists at times revealed such factual information as their levels of training as well as more personal information such as their motivations for conducting the group therapy and their emotional reactions to what the clients reported. The therapists did not at any time self-disclose personal problems, concerns, or past experiences.

Therapists' training. When the UCLA project began, other treatment programs for clients who had experienced sexual intimacy with their previous therapists also were just in their infancy. The staff then did not know from anyone's experience what clinical issues were likely to emerge. Following the completion of the first group, four members of the UCLA project (Sonne et al. 1985) reported three major clinical issues that surfaced repeatedly for clients in the group treatment: difficulties with trust, impaired self-concept, and problems in expressing anger. A second paper published in 1986 further elaborated these problem areas (Borys et al. 1986). Increasing exchange among professionals concerned with this clinical population validated the generality of the presenting clinical issues. Therapists who are planning to offer group treatment to clients who have experienced sexual intimacy with a therapist would be well advised to familiarize

themselves with these issues, briefly summarized below (for additional reference material, see also Kaufman and Harrison 1986;
Luepker and Retsch-Bogard 1986; Pope and Bouhoutsos 1986).

Professionals appear to agree that the most critical and central
issue for victims of sexual intimacy in therapy is their profound and
generalized mistrust of others. This mistrust is not surprising given
the betrayal experienced by clients when professionals to whom they
have turned for help with the most intimate concerns actually abused
them psychologically, and in some cases, physically. Clients then
enter group therapy with considerable suspicion of the group therapists, and their primary concern is whether this therapy also will
involve sexual intimacy. Project therapists assured clients from the
outset that sexual intimacy in the therapeutic context is illegal and
unethical and would not occur in the group. Indeed, the degree to
which any physical contact (such as a handshake or a touch on the
back) would take place was discussed and left to each client's prefer-
ence.

The second area of suspicion that emerges regards the therapists'
competency and motivation. Project clients were wary of why the
therapists began such a group and why the therapists requested certain procedures within the group. Clients' underlying concern appeared to be the fear that therapists would, at some point, act in their
own best interest, ignoring the clients' welfare.

Clients' mistrust extends beyond the new therapists to the other
group members, to professional institutions, and to significant others
in their lives. And, in addition to mistrusting others, the clients appear
to mistrust themselves. Understandably, they question their own perceptions, motives, and capacities to set limits in relationships. They
wonder how they could have depended on and sacrificed for therapists who eventually betrayed them.

Clinicians have also noted marked self-concept impairment in
clients who have experienced sexual intimacy in therapy. In the PTSP
groups, the impairment was evident in four areas: low self-esteem,
heightened dependency, desire for specialness, and sexuality. Self-
deprecation and self-blame for the involvement with the therapist was
common. Many clients expressed feelings of powerlessness and
incompetency that heightened their sense of dependency on others,
including the therapists in the group treatment. Further, many of the
clients mourned the loss of feeling special, truly loved by the former
therapist. Finally, clients expressed a cautiousness or even disgust
with their sexual impulses and behavior as a result of sexual involve-

ment with their previous therapists. For some female clients who identified themselves as heterosexual before they were involved sexually with female therapists, there tended to be significant confusion over their "true" sexual orientation.

Direct expression of anger appears problematic whether directed toward previous therapists, new group therapists, other group members, or significant others. PTSP clients tended to fear that their anger at their former therapist could be overwhelming should it begin to surface. Most angry feelings, then, tended to be defended against and ultimately were expressed through fantasies and dreams, nonverbal behavior, or intellectualized discussion.

Planning and debriefing sessions.   Planning and debriefing sessions for the cotherapists, supervisors, and project staff were held around each PTSP group session. Although at times the sessions felt tedious, their value was unquestionable. A 30-minute planning meeting before the group session allowed the cotherapists to apprise each other of important information gathered over the week (e.g., if a client had contacted one of the therapists during the week), to recheck the overall treatment plan and individual session strategy, and to mutually anticipate any problems or issues that might arise in that night's group session. The debriefing session lasted approximately 1 hour after the group therapy session. It gave the cotherapists time to chart treatment notes and to discuss the content and process of the immediately preceding group with staff consultants, to address special problems that required particular action by a cotherapist before the next group (e.g., call an absent group member), and to discuss transference and countertransference issues.

GROUP MEMBER SELECTION PROCESS AND CRITERIA

Intake interview.   As stated at the beginning of this chapter, prospective PTSP group members had responded to newspaper articles, public announcements, and professional and personal referrals. Project staff asked respondents to come to the UCLA Psychology Clinic for an intake interview. The purpose of the intake interview was threefold: to assess each client's need and suitability for group psychotherapy, to give information regarding the nature of the group, and to build rapport with the prospective clients.

During the intake interview, a PTSP staff member obtained information about the client's interest in the group, the current life situation, a brief description of the client's relationship and sexual involvement with the previous therapist, and a history of psychological status since the sexual involvement, including depression, suicidal ideation or attempts, psychiatric hospitalizations, loss of marriage or other important relationships, and drug or alcohol abuse. Although it was usual that one of the PTSP group leaders conducted the initial interview, Luepker and Retsch-Bogard (1986) suggest that it is more advantageous to have both leaders present for all intakes.

The intake staff also administered an MMPI to each prospective client during the intake session. Clearly, there were advantages and disadvantages to such a formal assessment. The major advantage was the access to clients' psychological status at that time. The main disadvantage was that the formal assessment was perceived by some clients to be a process through which the staff could indirectly find out something about them, something that they may not know or want revealed. Clients felt scrutinized and evaluated. To help alleviate these feelings, PTSP staff gave each interviewee a formal feedback session to discuss the assessment findings. However, the feelings persisted for some individuals. In one PTSP treatment group, the group members asked the group leaders to take an MMPI to prove their "fitness" for leading the group just as they had had to prove theirs for joining it.

During the intake interview, the intake staff also described the structure, function, and parameters of the group treatment. Expectations for attendance, cancellation procedures, and fee requirements were discussed as well.

Third, and perhaps most importantly, the intake staff engaged in initial rapport building with the prospective client during the first session. The interviewer's clarity, openness, and unconditional acceptance of the client appeared to ease the transition toward this goal. The interviewer emphasized that the group sessions would provide clients with a safe, nonjudgmental, confidential environment in which they would be encouraged, but not coerced, to share their experiences and their feelings.

Inclusion/exclusion criteria. The most critical criterion for the inclusion of specific clients in a PTSP group was evidence of their positive motivation to participate in the group treatment after the intake interview. The project staff had formulated some exclusion criteria before beginning the first group. Clients who evidenced acute psychosis or severe depression with acute suicidal ideation and recent attempt(s) were considered not likely to be good candidates for group therapy. However, the staff actually had to dissuade very few from group treatment based on these criteria. When such a decision was made, the staff made every effort to ensure that these clients who were asked not to participate had access to more appropriate treatment resources, specifically individual therapy with a clinician experienced with the issues associated with therapist-client sexual intimacy.

It is important to note that while project staff did not exclude many prospective clients from group treatment, many clients were ambivalent about joining after the intake interview, and several chose not to participate. The ambivalence and resistance evident is most likely reflective of the understandable and generalized mistrust of therapy. Some of these clients expressed a willingness to pursue individual therapy. However, some were unlikely to engage in any treatment at that time, even though in need.

GROUP PROCESS ISSUES

Three major group process issues emerged repeatedly in the PTSP group treatment of clients who had experienced sexual intimacy with their former therapists: confidentiality/privilege issues, boundary issues, and therapist countertransference issues.

Confidentiality/privilege. Predictably, clients entered group treatment with tremendous concern about the privacy of what they might reveal within the group. These clients had suffered great violations of trust by their former therapists and, in many cases, violations of the ethical limits of confidentiality and legal limits of privilege as well. It was imperative that the group leaders initiate a full and open discussion of the clients' ethical and legal rights to privacy and any limitations to those rights. For instance, clients were informed that if they initiated legal proceedings against the former therapists, privilege in current and past therapy generally would be waived automatically. Thus, the group therapists could be subpoenaed to testify in court and asked to reveal information regarding the clients and current treatment.

The PTSP staff was also aware that legal proceedings could bring a specific client to the attention of the media, which might pursue access to the group treatment facility and staff. The project staff needed to reiterate clearly their ethical and legal responsibilities to protect each client's privacy.

Group therapists also discussed with the group the process of record keeping (charting) and what personnel would have access to the records. The group leaders were aware that records could be subpoenaed and thus could be a source of information read by possibly antagonistic persons not trained in mental health. Notes were written clearly and with discretion. Names and other identifying information of other group participants were not entered into individual charts.

Third, the group leaders discussed the possibility of their consultation with adjunct psychotherapy, medical, or legal supports for any individual client. The occasion of the consultation and the specific information revealed about clients was released formally in writing by clients after they had been informed fully. Again therapists were aware of the limitations of the clients' privilege and presented those limitations clearly to the group.

The PTSP clients reviewed and individually signed confidentiality contracts explicitly stating that they would refrain from talking about the group participants or discussions to persons outside the group or among themselves in a public place where they could be overheard. One group requested that the therapists sign the same document (which they did). The clients also decided whether they would reveal the names of the offending therapists within the group discussions. Many clients suspected a type of collegial allegiance that could be invoked if the group therapists knew one of the offending therapists.

Boundaries. The majority of clients involved in group treatment following sexual intimacy with a former therapist experienced difficulties with the negotiation of interpersonal boundaries in the group. These difficulties appeared to stem primarily from the ambivalence the clients felt toward therapeutic relationships. On one hand, clients typically recognized their vulnerability, their need for help, and their desire for nurturance. On the other hand, they feared the loss of their control and objectivity, and, ultimately, the sense of personal identity should they trust the group therapist and other group members with those needs and desires.

Reflective of this ambivalence, clients requested longer group sessions and sought extended involvement with the therapists and other group members outside of the group context, including phone calls during the week, dinner invitations, and discussions in the hallways of the clinic. Yet within the group sessions, clients were likely to evidence a reluctance to self-disclose or to display much assertion or activity. Many clients appeared quite sensitive to even low-level interpretation of what they presented by the therapists or other members. Physical touching intended to comfort or support was viewed as very threatening by many members.

The group therapist, then, was confronted with the complex task of helping clients determine and set appropriate interpersonal boundaries. Modeling by the therapists appeared to be very helpful. As the group leaders limited intrusions into the boundaries of the therapeutic relationship (e.g., declined a dinner invitation) and displayed and encouraged appropriate self-disclosure within the group process, group members typically expressed relief with the clarity of boundaries and began to negotiate more actively their own.

Countertransference.   The third group process issue focuses more specifically on the therapists' reactions rather than the clients'. Therapists' countertransference with clients who have been sexually intimate with a former therapist is a powerful and complex phenomenon. A predominant countertransference reaction for the PTSP therapists was a desire to be the "perfect" therapist to right the egregious wrong of the previous therapist and help the victim. Several dangers were inherent in this type of reaction. First, the reaction encouraged a sense that the clinicians needed to be very careful not to make any mistakes. From this sense of carefulness, the therapists tended to become more self-aware rather than more oriented toward the clients. As a result, the therapists felt less observant and understanding of the clients at times. Second, occasionally therapists were inclined to become overly indulgent and to forgo interpretations or limit setting that might upset or anger clients.

A second countertransference reaction for the PTSP therapists was the experience of outrage toward the offending therapist, for harming the client and for besmirching the profession. Therapists' anger, if not analyzed and controlled, could have interfered with clients' therapy in several ways. Most importantly, if clients recognized the therapists' anger, they may have felt pressure to pursue their own anger in group therapy and suppress or repress the other side of the ambivalent feelings experienced toward the offending therapist. Many clients continued to admire and care for their previous therapists for a long time after the intimacy. Moreover, angry group therapists might have forcefully "encouraged" the clients to seek redress through legal and/or ethical channels. Formal ethical or legal complaints typically involve clients in long and taxing processes, often too arduous even for those clients who begin the process on their own initiative. And finally, the group therapists may have actively or even subtly devalued the offending therapist, which may have encouraged maladaptive splitting, rather than the integration of the client's positive and negative feelings toward the previous clinician.

A third countertransference reaction involved the PTSP therapists' discomfort with, and even resentment of, the potential or actual demands of the group members. Most clinicians who have worked with this client population recognize the vulnerability and complexity of the clients, making the treatment difficult and taxing. However, the therapists' efforts to help frequently end in rejection by the clients because of their mistrust of and anger with therapy. Borys et al. (1986) suggest that familiarity with the management of similar countertransference issues in the treatment of the borderline patient (e.g., Briggs 1979; Kernberg 1975) may help group therapists work through the reaction.

As mentioned earlier in the chapter, the debriefing sessions for the therapists and PTSP staff following the group treatment proved to be invaluable in the recognition and handling of the countertransference reactions.

TERMINATION ISSUES

Termination of the PTSP treatment groups proved to be difficult, even though the time-limited parameter of the groups was stated and restated. The difficulty was undoubtedly due in part to the fact that the terminations with offending therapists were most often abrupt and countertherapeutic, and clients were typically left with unresolved feelings of abandonment, devastation, and rage. Termination of the PTSP group then not only raised issues of separation from the group but also re-evoked unresolved previous termination reactions.

OUTCOME

In our experience, group therapy for victims of therapist-client intimacy proved to be an effective and helpful, albeit complex, intervention. Clients have reported that the group provided them with a much-needed place to share their disturbing experiences and the emotional and cognitive upset related to those experiences. Participants felt acknowledged and supported. All of the clients acknowledged that they had benefited from the group therapy. The group experience appeared specifically helpful for all clients in alleviating 5 of the 10 major aspects of Pope's therapist-patient sex syndrome presented in Chapter 4: emptiness and isolation, guilt, emotional lability or dyscontrol, increased suicidal risk, and cognitive dysfunction (i.e., flashbacks, intrusive thoughts, nightmares). Improvement in the 5 other aspects (impaired ability to trust, ambivalence, suppressed rage, sexual confusion, and identity and role reversal) tended to be more dependent on the specific dynamics of the individual client.

Clients who struggled with continuing and intense issues of mistrust and ambivalence were least likely to benefit from the group and tended to be most disruptive of effective group process. While group cohesion was difficult to establish initially because of most of the participants' generalized mistrust of the new therapists and the other group members, it was further impeded as time went on when a few clients continued an intense inability to trust. Without solid group cohesion, critical issues could not be explored in depth. Also, as a result of their continuing ambivalent idealization of the former therapists, some clients struggled within the group process to regain the sense of "specialness" once experienced in the sexualized therapeutic relationship. Rivalry for the group leaders' attention proved disruptive to the group process. Individual therapy prior to the group therapy, or at least concomitant with group therapy, is highly advisable for this type of client.

In light of the fact that therapist-client sexual intimacy does occur with alarming frequency, with often devastating effects on clients, mental health professionals must focus their efforts to effectively treat the victims and move toward prevention of the intimacy. Graduate and continuing education for mental health professionals need increased recognition and discussion of the problem. Finally, empirical research must begin to keep pace with the rapidly growing clinical literature on therapist-client sexual intimacy.

Chapter 9

Sexual Intimacies After Termination: Clinical, Ethical, and Legal Aspects

Glen O. Gabbard, M.D.
Kenneth S. Pope, Ph.D.

The facts presented in this volume form a disturbing picture. It is clear that sexual intimacies between therapists and those with whom they form a professional relationship are harmful and can, in fact, be devastating.

It is also clear that a dismaying number of professionals (perhaps 10 percent of male therapists) engage in this practice and use a variety of rationalizations. Some claim that such intimacies cannot be prohibited by any professional organization, governmental entity, or ethical code. Uncoerced activities occurring in private between adults, they argue, are always legitimate (an argument that would permit therapist-patient sex both before and after termination). Others claim that such intimacies are safe and legitimate as long as they are not presented as part of treatment. Still others claim to have discovered a "safe area" in which the characteristic harm does not occur (e.g., sex occurring in the context of "true love," sex occurring outside of the therapist's office, sex occurring between—rather than during—sessions, sex occurring after termination).

There are, of course, fallacies embodied in each of these claims. In this chapter, we will focus on only one of these claims, namely, that after termination, ethical prohibitions no longer apply. The reasons that termination does not legitimize or make safe sexual intimacy with a patient are many. We will highlight a few.

TRANSFERENCE

All therapeutic situations are colored to some degree by transference. The patient begins to experience the therapist as though he or she were a parent, and therefore erotic feelings in the transference are symbolically incestuous (Barnhouse 1978). The reasons that the therapist does not respond to the erotic feelings of the patient (or to his or her own erotic countertransference) were eloquently stated by Freud (1915):

> If the patient's advances were returned it would be a great triumph for her, but a complete defeat for the treatment. She would have succeeded in what all patients strive for in analysis—she would have succeeded in acting out, in repeating in real life, what she ought only to have remembered, to have reproduced as psychical material and to have kept within the sphere of psychical events. In the further course of the love-relationship, she would bring out all the inhibitions and pathological reactions of her erotic life, without there being any possibility of correcting them; and the distressing episode would end in remorse and a great strengthening of her propensity to repression. The love-relationship in fact destroys the patient's susceptibility to influence from analytic treatment. (p. 166)

To rationalize the acceptability of sex with patients after termination, one would need to demonstrate that transference no longer exists after termination of treatment. However, the facts are otherwise. The transference is never fully resolved. Even in formal analysis, where detailed interpretation of the transference neurosis constitutes the cornerstone of treatment, transference residues of varying intensity always remain. Pfeffer's (1963) follow-up study of patients after termination found that even well-analyzed patients easily regress and revive the transference paradigms that were typical of their analyses. He concluded: "After the analysis, the patient retains an important and complicated intrapsychic representation of the analyst" (p. 230). Similarly, Norman et al.'s (1976) follow-up studies 2 or more years after termination of an analysis deemed successful by both therapist and patient found that "the transference neurosis remains as a latent structure" (p. 496). Oremland et al. (1975) noted that patients typically carry an unanalyzed idea of the analyst with them even after termination. Carlson's (1986) study of patient dreams after termination of psychotherapy concluded that "transference phenomena are implicated in posttreatment consolidation of experience" (p. 251). These studies suggest that should either the therapist or the patient approach the other and enter into a sexually intimate relationship, the transference situation itself would be instantly reactivated and intensified, and whatever posttermination consolidation, working through, and reexamination was occurring would be thwarted.

Moreover, a sexual consummation of this sort may correspond precisely with the unresolved transference wish of the patient. Calef and Weinshel (1983) report that it is common for patients to terminate with a feeling of "unfinished business." This feeling often relates to the patient's sexual wishes to consummate the relationship with the analyst at some time. The authors note that this feeling may be present in patients who are otherwise well analyzed. Such longings for consummation—longings which, as Freud stressed, must remain on the psychical level and never be acted out on the physical level—may persist for many years after termination.

The unresolved transference that remains after termination is by no means limited to patients in psychoanalysis. Buckley et al. (1981), for example, studied the effects of psychotherapy as well as psychoanalysis. Their subjects were 97 psychotherapists preselected by virtue of having completed therapy or analysis. Their research, conducted at Albert Einstein College of Medicine, suggests that "a gradual working through of unresolved transference issues with the passage of time following the treatment" (p. 304) may be an important determinant of successful therapy:

> Analysis of the data also revealed that thoughts about the therapist reach a peak during the 5–10-year period following treatment. . . . All of the respondents in the 5–10-year period following therapy reported experiencing thoughts of returning to analysis or therapy. This would seem to be a critical time in the post-therapeutic development. (p. 304)

There seem to be no research data to demonstrate that transference disappears or even begins to lessen in intensity upon termination. The data that do exist seem to indicate that the "transference residue" in psychotherapy and psychoanalysis in fact peaks during the period between 5 and 10 years after termination.

Herman et al. (1987; see also Brodsky 1988 and Ethics Committee of the American Psychological Association 1988), reviewing their national study of sexual intimacies between psychiatrists and their therapy patients, affirm the view that transference does not end with the termination of the face-to-face therapeutic sessions. They point out that the concept of a supposed "waiting period" after termination before sexual intimacies are initiated is naïve because it does not take into account the timeless nature of the unconscious. The intrapsychic attachments to incestuous figures, whether parents or therapists, know no time limits.

The taboo is never broken. While different schools of psychotherapy approach transference differently, this taboo is inviolable regardless of theoretical orientation. In the case of psychoanalytically oriented therapy, the very essence of the treatment is that the patient must ultimately give up incestuous childhood wishes. One must mourn their loss so that one can get on with one's life and develop more mature and appropriate object relatedness. If there is any doubt in the patient's mind, he or she may postpone this grief work and hold on to the fantasy that someday such wishes will be gratified.

To argue that the taboo against therapist-patient sexual relations can be broken at some future date in the course of any therapeutic approach would be just as absurd as an argument suggesting that the taboo against parent-offspring sexual relations can be broken once the child has grown up, has left home, is independent and knowledgeable, and has the right, as an adult, to give informed consent to a sexual relationship with any other adult, including a parent.

THE INTERNALIZED THERAPIST

The transference, by definition, is unconscious and represents a distortion. The patient reacts to the therapist as if the therapist were an important figure from the patient's past. During the course of the therapeutic sessions and after termination, the transference must be handled in one of two ways if the therapy is to be effective. First, in some therapies (or phases of some therapies), the transference itself is not analyzed. Rather it is "managed," either by attempting to keep it from interfering with the therapeutic work or by harnessing it in service of the therapeutic work (as in so-called "transference cures"). Second, in some therapies, and certainly in psychoanalysis, the transference is analyzed. In other words, through interpretation patients become aware of how they are reacting to the therapist as if the therapist were a figure from the past, accompanied by all the feelings and conflicts associated with that figure.

Yet the transferential attachment to the therapist (i.e., an internal representation of the therapist, which is unconscious and which involves fundamental distortions) is but one way in which the patient internalizes an "image" of the therapist. Other internal representations need not involve transference, can be both conscious and realistic (i.e., free of significant distortion), and tend to play a crucial role in the therapy, both prior to and after termination of the therapeutic sessions themselves. In fact, they are in large part responsible for the continuation of the beneficial effects of therapy after the cessation of the sessions. As Edelson (1963) put it:

> The problem of termination is not how to get therapy stopped, or when to stop it, but how to terminate so that what has been happening keeps on "going" inside the patient. The problem of termination is not simply one of helping the patient to achieve independence in the sense of willingness to function in the physical absence of the therapist. More basically it is a problem of facilitating achievement by the patient of the ability to "hang on" to the therapist (or the experience of the relationship with the therapist) *in his physical absence* in the form of a realistic intrapsychic representation (memories, identification—associated with altered functioning) which is conserved rather than destructively or vengefully abandoned following separation, thus making mastery of this experience possible. (p. 14)

Research conducted by Geller et al. (1981–82) at Yale University studied the ways in which hundreds of individuals "create and interpret mental representations of their therapists and the psychotherapeutic process both during therapy and after termination" (p. 123). Examples of common aspects of these mental representations—some of which are not transference based, while others are clearly influenced by transference distortions—include:

> "When I am faced with a difficult situation I sometimes ask myself, 'What would my therapist do?' "
> "In a sense, I feel as though my therapist has become a part of me."
> "I try to solve my problems in the way my therapist and I worked on them in psychotherapy."
> "I wish I could be friends with my therapist."
> "I wonder if my therapist ever thinks about me."
> "I imagine being held by my therapist."
> "I imagine having sex with my therapist."
> "I miss my therapist."

"I daydream about my therapist."
"I think about contacting my therapist."
"I imagine our kissing each other."
"I miss talking about myself the way therapy permits me to do."
"I imagine a particular quality to the sound of my therapist's voice."
"I imagine my therapist sitting in his/her office."
"I picture a specific expression on my therapist's face."
"I am aware of a particular emotional atmosphere which gives me the sense that my therapist is 'with me.' "
"I doubt that anyone can replace my therapist in my life."

Factor analyses of the data allowed exploration of interrelationships among the stylistic, functional, and formal properties of such internalized representations across different states of consciousness and in different situations. Among the findings was the fact that "the vividness of the representation and the use of the representation for the purpose of continuing the therapeutic dialogue are significantly correlated with self-perceived improvement" (p. 123). Thus the internalized "images" of the therapist appear to continue after termination and to play a significant role in the effectiveness of the therapy.

Continuing Professional Responsibilities

The professional relationship between therapist and patient exists past termination in other ways besides the transference and the realistic intrapsychic representations. Formal ethical standards, legislation, and case law establishing that the therapist is obligated to respond appropriately to the patient's rights to privacy, confidentiality, and privilege (three separate though interrelated concepts), and that this obligation is unaffected by termination or the passage of time after termination, is but one form of recognition that the professional relationship does not dissolve and vanish upon the ceasing of the therapy sessions. Similarly, most states have passed legislation requiring therapists to maintain records beyond the date of termination. When served with a valid subpoena (e.g., the privilege has been waived either directly through consent of the patient or indirectly through certain actions or circumstances of the patient), the therapist cannot refuse to offer expert testimony concerning his or her assessment of the patient's prior mental status and response to treatment, for example, simply because the therapy sessions have been terminated.

Such professional responsibilities are manifestations of important aspects of the professional relationship that persist once the therapy has been initiated and despite termination. To deny the continuing existence of the professional relationship in order to engage in sexual intimacies with a patient after termination is contrary to these facts.

In addition to these legal/ethical/professional reasons, there is also a practical clinical reason to assume continuing professional responsibilities for the patient. He or she may return for more treatment. In a recent study of 71 successfully analyzed patients, two-thirds of them had recontacted their analysts within 3 years of termination (Hartlaub et al. 1986). These patients did not return because their analyses were incomplete and ineffective. On the contrary, they were doing rather well, but required a few more consultations to solidify the gains they had made in their analyses. Some, for example, needed to work on the continued de-idealization of the analyst, further evidence of the continuation of transference issues after termination. Others needed assistance in reactivating their own self-analytic function. Still others felt the need to report developmentally important accomplishments and thereby continue the process of restructuring internal self- and object-representations.

UNEQUAL POWER

The distorted transferential reactions, the realistic intrapsychic representations, and the aspects of the formal professional relationship, all of which endure past the termination of the therapy sessions, indicate that—however much therapists may wish to conceal, discount, or deny it—there is a profound power differential between therapists and their patients, regardless of termination.

One aspect of this power differential is what may be called the "blackmail" power of the therapist. Even in sexual relationships in which the power differential is not as pronounced as that which occurs between therapist and patient, one partner may take unfair advantage of the other. Women, for instance, may experience "date rape" or various forms of physical abuse. Ultimately, victims of such exploitation may need to press a complaint in civil and/or criminal court, either to be "made whole" for prior suffering or to gain protection from future attacks. But a woman who has been a patient of a sexual partner may face a formidable obstacle in placing her mental and emotional state at issue before courts of any kind, for such action may be equivalent to waiving her rights to confidentiality and privilege. Thus her sexual partner, who was once her therapist, may discount her complaint and use as evidence material from her therapy. Anything she may have said in therapy, as well as any professional opinions the therapist may wish to assert in defending himself, may become part of a public record or of newspaper accounts. The most private aspects of her life—as interpreted through the "authoritative" eyes of a sexual partner against whom she has filed a complaint—may become public. In so many ways, the power differential and the patient's vulnerability persist regardless of the termination of the therapy sessions.

It should be noted that some therapists within certain theoretical orientations (e.g., humanistic, feminist) aspire to a therapy in which there is no power differential whatsoever, in which status, authority, roles, and all aspects of power are completely equal. For such approaches to be seen as possibly justifying therapist-client sexual intimacies, they would need to achieve their aspirations in actuality. As a bare minimum, in such a relationship, neither of the two people would work under a title (e.g., therapist) or a state investment of authority (e.g., a license) not available to the other, neither would have a unique authority to assign a diagnosis (for insurance or other purposes) to the other, and—most important—a power imbalance could never be created through one paying money to the other.

THE HARM BOTH TO PATIENTS AND
TO THE THERAPY PROCESS

If posttermination sexual intimacies between therapists and patients were to become legitimized, the therapeutic process as we know it would drastically change. Therapists, patients, and potential patients would all come to understand that a sexual relationship between the therapist and patient is a possibility for some patients, if not immediately at termination, then somewhere down the line, and that this is a legitimate outcome.

Patients experiencing the sexual attraction common to transference could discard the "outmoded" concept of trying to analyze this phenomenon in the safety of a "holding environment," and instead begin working on what may seem a much more pressing concern: how to ensure that the sexual union will actually take place once the termination is out of the way. Looking attractive may be important. Pleasing—and perhaps sexually teasing—the therapist may play a role. Not mentioning material about which one is ashamed or embarrassed may be crucial, since it may cause the therapist to see one in an unfavorable and less sexually desirable light. Not bringing up uncomfortable and troublesome thoughts and feelings that would tend to prolong the course of therapy, and thus delay the gratification of the hoped-for posttermination sexual intimacies, would be a fundamental rule. In fact, eager patients may simply decide to terminate the therapy sessions promptly, with or without the concurrence of the therapist, so that the prohibition against sex will become inactive sooner.

Other changes may be somewhat less apparent. Because the patient knows that the possibility of a posttermination sexual union is not at all prohibited, and because the therapist seems so desirable, it may seem less important, perhaps even counterproductive, to attempt to examine, improve, or otherwise change the current relationships the patient has in his or her life.

It is extremely common for patients to experience an intense desire to be their therapist's "favorite" patient. Many patients feel jealousy (and relive sibling rivalries) toward other patients, real or imagined. If posttermination therapist-patient sexual intimacies were ever accepted as legitimate by the professions, patients would be provided a specific arena in which to compete for favored status.

Therapists would be free to use their practices as an ideal dating service. What better way to screen potential sexual partners and to find out the most intimate details about their sexual history, their personalities, their habits, their incomes, and their expectations—and to get paid for it! Patients become fair game, and every time a "winner" turns up, once the therapist is ready to make his or her move (having waited until termination and any appropriate additional period), he or she knows the vulnerabilities and the likes and dislikes of the patient. It would even be possible that therapists would begin to compare notes and to compete among themselves to make sure that they "bag the limit," in the same way that some professors seem to enjoy sexual encounters with either the largest number of or the most attractive students and seem to enjoy sharing their exploits with each other (see Chapter 13).

Thus legitimizing posttermination intimacies would affect both patients who might desire sexual intimacy with their therapist and therapists who might desire sexual intimacy with their patients. But it would also affect patients who did not desire such a relationship. Those who feel guilty, anxious, ashamed, embarrassed, or concerned over aspects of their own sexuality may wonder if their disclosures will prompt the therapist to give them a posttermination call for dinner and drinks. Rape victims may wonder if their accounts of the experience are being responded to solely on the professional level. Incest victims who have grown to fear that even a seemingly safe relationship may become sexualized may wonder what the therapist is planning. Patients who have presenting problems often termed "Don Juanism" or nymphomania, as well as those who bemoan the fact that they have a hard time saying "no," may find their therapist paying inordinate attention to them, and copying their phone number from the chart into a black book. Any patient may wonder when the therapist may suddenly suggest the termination of therapy, perhaps for other than therapeutic reasons.

Finally, not only would the patient's current therapy process be subverted, but future therapy processes would be destroyed. How would the patient be able to trust the next therapist after becoming disillusioned with a posttermination relationship? Why should they believe that the therapist would sincerely put a patient's interests as primary? Such concerns could not be dealt with as pure fantasy since there would be an obvious basis for them in reality. The trust in the therapist, so essential for the development of a therapeutic alliance, would be irreparably damaged.

LEGISLATION

In considering the possible consequences of legitimizing post-termination sexual intimacies, it is important to maintain awareness that what is "legal" is not necessarily moral, ethical, and good practice. All too frequently, politicians and others who are challenged on ethical and moral grounds defend the most destructive, unethical, and immoral acts as "technically not a violation of the law."

Nevertheless, states have been initiating more and more specific legislation to protect patients against exploitation before and after termination. The firmest leadership has been provided by the state of Florida. Chapter 21U-15.004 states: "For purposes of determining the existence of sexual misconduct as defined herein, the psychologist-client relationship is deemed to continue in perpetuity."

Even California, not known for strict views or standards in regard to sexual activities, currently has in force Civic Code section 43.93, which sets forth a cause of action for a patient or former patient to recover damages from a therapist who engages in sexual contact with the patient or former patient "within 2 years following psychotherapy."

THE SELF-INTEREST OF RISK MANAGEMENT

Those therapists finding themselves overwhelmed by sexual interest in a patient, undeterred by the considerations outlined thus far (which focus on the well-being and protection of the patient), and contemplating a posttermination coupling, may at least want to consider the risks to themselves. Posttermination sexual relationships seem to be lacking in endorsement by civil courts, licensing boards, and ethics committees. Thus a complaint by the patient or third party to one of these agencies may call the therapist to account, and the accounting may involve a financial judgment, suspension or loss of license, and censure by or expulsion from the professional association.

Tempted therapists may wish to read the case of *Whitesell* v. *Green* [No. 38745, Dist. Ct. Hawaii filed November 19, 1973] in which the court held that termination did not legitimize a therapist's later sexual involvement with a patient.

They may wish to consider Sell et al.'s (1986) multiyear study of state licensing boards and state ethics committees. The study found "that psychologists asserting that a sexual relationship had occurred only after the termination of the therapeutic relationship were more likely to be found in violation than those not making that claim" (p. 504).

They may wish to take into account the case reported by the ethics committee of the American Psychiatric Association (Recent ethics cases 1982) in which a psychiatrist argued that because the sexual relationship with the patient did not begin until a substantial time after the termination of the therapy, "the sexual activity took place outside the context of the doctor-patient relationship and was not unethical" (p. 9). The district branch of the American Psychiatric Association Ethics Committee, however, held that the "timing of the commencement of the sexual relationship was not relevant. Even if the sexual activity did not start until after the termination of therapy, the psychiatrist's sexual involvement with the patient constituted exploitation of the 'knowledge, power and unique position that [the doctor] held in the patient's mental life,' so the district branch decided to *expel* the member-psychiatrist" (p. 9). The member-psychiatrist appealed the decision. However, the American Psychiatric Association Board of Trustees, upon recommendation of the American Psychiatric Association Ethics Committee, approved the action taken by the district branch. Since that decision, the Assembly of the American Psychiatric Association has approved a proposal that would make it explicitly unethical for psychiatrists to engage in sexual relations with former patients.

Those therapists still overwhelmed with temptation may wish to review their professional liability policies, especially the sections showing that the limitations in coverage regarding therapist-patient sexual intimacies apply to former as well as current patients.

They may wish to verify for themselves that there have been no published research studies demonstrating or even suggesting that therapist-patient sexual involvement becomes safe at a point 3 months or even 3 years after termination.

They may wish to note ethics texts—which may be introduced as evidence of expert opinion regarding sexual intimacies with patients after termination—that contain clear statements of the prohibition against becoming sexually involved with patients prior to or after termination. Dyer (1988), for example, summarizes his discussion of "the most *un*ambiguous point": "The prohibition about sex with patients (and of course former patients since transferences endure in time) is of crucial importance" (pp. 33–34).

They may want to take note of the views of their colleagues, a majority of whom condemn the practice. Close to two-thirds of a national sample of psychiatrists viewed the practice as an unequivocal breach of ethics (Herman et al. 1987). Two-thirds of a national sample of psychologists found that posttermination sex was, under any and all circumstances, a violation of good standards of practice (Pope et al. 1988).

Tempted therapists desperate to justify their actions and finding no other available means, may attempt to use the concept of marriage. After all, could their motives or the consequences of their actions be questioned if they were considering marriage? Use of the institution of marriage to cloak or discount abuse and exploitation has a long and dishonorable tradition. For decades, physical assaults which would land a person in jail if the victim were a stranger or neighbor were ignored by law enforcement personnel and considered acceptable by many (including, not infrequently, both spouses) if they were "merely" cases of spouse abuse. A frequent component of the battered spouse syndrome—which bears similarities to therapist-patient sex syndrome—is that the victim often feels that she (and the victim usually is a "she") provokes and deserves the beatings, that she is truly fortunate to be involved with such a wonderful man, and that there is nothing "out of the ordinary" about such activity.

Similarly, rape has been for many years considered by law and by custom as "justified" and "natural" when occurring in the context of marriage. Or, put another way, rape was considered impossible within the context of marriage. It was as if the very mention of the word marriage masked the real sexual exploitation that was occurring. To those who doubted the legitimacy of such rapes, it was pointed out that frequently the supposedly abused spouse remained in the marriage, not only failing to make a complaint but often defending her husband.

Only gradually are we changing our view that acts which are otherwise exploitative, abusive, and harmful are somehow legitimate, natural, and even healthy after a marriage ceremony. Finally, those who are still tempted and are unmoved by the appeals to self-interest and self-protection presented so far may wish to try one last selfish appeal: Consider how behaving with such disregard for the safety and well-being of your patient will make you feel. Can you harm your patient without harming your own integrity?

CONCLUSION

In this chapter we have outlined seven of the major reasons why sexual intimacies with patients after termination are clinically, ethically, and professionally unacceptable. Anyone wishing to justify sexual intimacies with patients—either before or after termination— needs to present clear and convincing evidence contradicting the reasons for the prohibition, including the seven outlined herein. Some individuals continue to assert that some forms of therapist-patient sexual intimacies are safe; for example, those which are not part of the treatment plan, those which occur outside of the therapy office, those which occur after termination, those which occur within certain theoretical orientations, those which occur with patients whose self-esteem or sexual functioning would somehow benefit from such intimacies, or those which do not occur during the therapy sessions. Until it is clear, contrary to the currently available evidence, that some forms of therapist-patient sexual intimacies are safe, therapist-patient sexual intimacies and the devastating harm that results must be avoided under all circumstances.

Chapter 10

Rehabilitation of Therapists Who Have Been Sexually Intimate with a Patient

Kenneth S. Pope, Ph.D.

Like the issue of whether incestuous parents should be allowed—by society, the courts, child protective services, and other family members—to resume the influential responsibilities for "parenting," the issue of whether therapists who engage in sexual contact with their patients should be authorized or recognized—by society, licensing boards, professional organizations, and prospective patients—as willing and able to resume clinical responsibilities is not yet settled. What seems clear, however, is that if certain matters are not addressed in an attempt at rehabilitation, it cannot be considered complete, and patients are once again placed at risk for great and lasting harm.

The purpose of this chapter is to outline the basic steps that are necessary (whether or not all would agree that they are sufficient) in preparing therapists to return to practice.

AVOIDING DUAL ROLES, BIAS, AND CONFLICTS OF INTEREST

For efforts at rehabilitation to have both the appearance and the reality of legitimacy, it is necessary to ensure that role confusion, bias, and conflicts of interest are eliminated as far as possible.

Importance of the coordinator.   One person needs to coordinate the work of rehabilitation. That individual must have access to all relevant information, documents, and individuals. Especially when several agencies (e.g., a licensing board, a professional association, and the clinic that employs the offending psychologist) are involved, the potential for "splitting" and for confused communications is great. Each agency may tend to assume that one of the other agencies is taking care of certain responsibilities. Each professional involved in the rehabilitation plan may be reluctant to express any reservations about the adequacy of the rehabilitation because he or she assumes that everyone else sees no problem. The process can become victim to what Janis (1972) called "groupthink." The coordinator must assume full responsibility for ensuring that the rehabilitation plan is comprehensive, that it is based upon the most complete information and documentation possible, and that it is being carried out carefully.

Clarifying the therapeutic and rehabilitative tasks.   Therapist-patient sexual contact is often construed as a dual relationship: The therapeutic relationship is confused with a sexual relationship. It is crucially important that rehabilitation efforts avoid confusion of relationships, roles, and tasks. Any careful rehabilitation plan involves two separate professions involved in two distinct relationships with the offending therapist. First, there is the professional serving as rehabilitation specialist, who will focus on the offending therapist's professional views, procedures, work setting, and methods of risk management, so that those factors that contribute to the offending therapist's sexual exploitation of patients can be eliminated or at least minimized. Second, there is the professional who will serve as the offending clinician's psychotherapist, who will focus on the personal life of the therapist. Just as incestuous parents and other child sex abusers possess developmental deficits and/or conflicts that put them at risk for harmful and inappropriate sexual relationships, so too do therapists who engage in sex with their patients apparently suffer from similar psychopathology.

Selection of individuals to carry out the rehabilitation plan.   In no case should agencies or individuals who have responsibility for an offending therapist "rubber-stamp" the therapist's choice of a supposedly qualified rehabilitation specialist or therapist. In order to avoid a legitimate and unbiased rehabilitation process, offending therapists are often tempted to set up their own plans—schemes that are little more than window dressing. Offenders show an almost uncanny knack for finding otherwise outstanding professionals who simply have no education, training, or experience to serve as rehabilitation specialists. Or they can find a friend with good credentials who will agree to a pro forma therapy or rehabilitation. Agencies understaffed and overburdened may be sorely tempted to accept such pseudorehabilitation processes. The following two fictional (but reality-based) vignettes illustrate how the bogus process operates:

Vignette 1: Dr. X has constructed an innovative psychological intervention whereby he can diagnose "tension areas" associated with neuropsychological imbalances simply by having his patient undress and by "palpating" her groin area for 20 or 30 minutes. He has collected a number of scientific articles that he maintains "lay the basis" for his diagnostic procedure. When one of his female patients complained that he had spent almost an hour rubbing her clitoris, the licensing board suspended his license. One requirement for the restoration of the license was a letter from a therapist stating that he no longer had any psychological conflicts that would put him at risk for masturbating his patients.

Immediately after the complaint was filed, Dr. X became a patient of a well-known psychiatrist who was unfamiliar with the theory, research, and professional area of therapist-patient sex. During therapy, Dr. X brought in the scientific articles and explained in detail his "breakthrough" procedures. His therapist agreed that the original complaint had been filed by a deeply disturbed patient as a result of her psychotic state. He also agreed that the diagnostic technique showed considerable promise and was only condemned by the licensing board because of the generally Victorian attitudes regarding sex so prevalent among mental health professionals. The offending therapist agreed to cease any behavior that would offend his less enlightened colleagues. His therapist then wrote a letter to the licensing board assuring them that Dr. X was at no risk whatsoever for the sexual molestation of patients. Dr. X's license was promptly restored, and he was able, for the next 4 years, to continue testing his innovative technique on his patients.

Vignette 2: The administrator of Freedonia Hospital was horrified when a patient presented him with clear evidence (including tape recordings, photographs, and handwritten letters from the doctor) that her therapist, Dr. Y, had been engaging in sexual intimacies with her. He promised to investigate. He called in Drs. A and B, who owned shares in the hospital and who were golfing partners of Dr. Y. The administrator asked them to "look into the matter." One week later, Dr. A filed a report indicating that the matter had been completely taken care of. The administrator met again with the patient and assured her that Dr. Y had received harsh and appropriate discipline and would never again be in a position to sexually abuse a patient. In this manner he was able to head off both a civil suit and a complaint to the licensing board. One year later, when another patient filed a complaint with the licensing board, Dr. Y was put on probation (rather than being suspended or having his license revoked) because he submitted letters from the administrator, Dr. A, and Dr. B attesting to the fact that Dr. Y had become aware of his problem long before this complaint was filed, had sought appropriate help (psychotherapy and rehabilitation from Drs. A and B), and was, in their professional opinion, now completely rehabilitated.

Without exception, legitimate rehabilitation plans consist of third parties (such as the licensing board or professional association) selecting potential rehabilitation specialists and therapists who meet all of the following criteria:

1. None of them is a friend or acquaintance of the offending therapist.
2. None of them shares any professional, business, economic, or similar relationship with the offending therapist (i.e., none works at the same hospital, sits on a committee with the offending therapist, teaches at the same medical or graduate school).
3. None of them has a record of significant legal or ethical violation.
4. All of them are knowledgeable about the area of therapist-patient sexual intimacy.

The third party may offer the offending therapist a list of three to five potential therapists and three to five potential rehabilitation specialists from which the offending therapist can choose those with whom to work.

Independent evaluation of the efficacy of the rehabilitation.   In many cases, a licensing board, a professional association, a hospital, or a clinic will want to determine whether an effort at rehabilitation has been effective. Should the individual's license be restored? Should the person's status as a "member in good standing" in the professional association be reinstated? Should a hospital or clinic hire the clinician and allow him or her to work with patients?

In such cases, the honest and detailed professional reports of both the offending clinician's therapist and the rehabilitation specialist will be invaluable. Both will have worked with the offending clinician over a long period of time and will have different perspectives from which they form their professional opinions. However, a different professional should conduct an independent evaluation to determine the extent to which the rehabilitation efforts have been effective. If, for instance, the rehabilitation specialist were to offer the final report he or she would, in essence, be attempting to evaluate his or her own efforts, and there is an inherent bias in such an evaluation. The independent professional must conduct a de novo assessment, utilizing direct clinical interviews with the offending clinician and the formal reports of both the rehabilitation specialist and the therapist. The various elements that this evaluation must address are presented in the following section.

ASSESSING THE ADEQUACY AND EFFECTIVENESS OF REHABILITATION

Those assuming the responsibility for evaluating whether an offending clinician has been adequately rehabilitated need to ensure that their deliberations and formal report address each of the following issues or aspects.

Depth and duration of the rehabilitation process. The offending clinician's formal work with both a therapist and a rehabilitation specialist must be of sufficient duration that genuine trust can develop, that the deep and often subtle and well-defended personality dynamics that lead to sexual abuse can emerge and be thoughtfully addressed, and that the complete spectrum of risks can be identified and minimized. One and one-half or 2 years is probably the minimum duration for the process to occur. As with incest, child sexual abuse, rape, and other forms of sexual abuse, the problems are not superficial, and the potential for continuing to engage in the behavior is great.

Coming to terms with the victim. The process of rehabilitation assumes that there has been at least one identified offense. Customarily, this offense comes to light when a patient files a complaint with the licensing board, a professional association, the treatment institution that employs the offending therapist, or the civil courts. An essential part of any genuine rehabilitation is that the offending therapist must work through and come to terms with the specific offense and with the harm done to this particular patient. Has the offending therapist acknowledged responsibility for sexually exploiting the patient? [In all cases and without exception, it is the therapist's responsibility to avoid sexual contact with a patient.] Has the offending therapist formally apologized to the patient? [For many patients, the offending therapist's direct acknowledgment and apology is a significant factor in the patient's recovery. It addresses many aspects of the damage that the patient may be experiencing—such as confusion, guilt, ambivalence—as described elsewhere in Chapter 4.] Has the offending therapist done all that is reasonable and within his or her power to diminish the damage and promote the recovery of the exploited patient? For many offending therapists, authentic rehabilitation does not begin until this initial necessary step is taken.

Formal reports of the rehabilitation specialist and therapist. To what extent are the reports provided by the offending clinician's therapist and rehabilitation specialist consistent and supplementary? If, taken together, they are confusing, contradictory, or incomplete, the professional conducting the evaluation needs to investigate further.

Records of all prior assessments and treatment. A careful and comprehensive assessment of the adequacy of rehabilitation efforts must include a review of all records of prior assessments and treatment. Often these documents (such as testing reports and chart notes) will reveal problems that, if unaddressed, set the stage for a new offense. Obtaining such records and reports will, of course, be possible only with the informed consent of the offending therapist.

Interviews with educators and employers. It is likely that the rehabilitation specialist—if he or she has developed a careful and comprehensive plan—has contacted the offending therapist's present and former teachers, clinical supervisors, employers, and administrative supervisors. However, in no case should a professional evaluating the adequacy of rehabilitation efforts submit a report without reliable information provided by those who have known the offending therapist professionally over the course of his or her development.

Reviewing any history of complaints. It may be that the offense that led to the current rehabilitation efforts was not the only one that has been identified. The relevant licensing boards and local, state, and national professional association and specialty boards should be contacted—with the informed consent of the offending clinician—to find out whether any complaints have been filed against the clinician and, if so, what the disposition of those complaints was.

Developmental history. As has been noted previously, sexually exploitative therapists, like incest perpetrators, child sexual abusers, and rapists, tend to show deficits or disturbances in their developmental histories. The personal therapy for offending clinicians, the rehabilitation work (e.g., discussions concerning countertransference), and the evaluation of the adequacy of rehabilitation efforts must all take serious and detailed account of the developmental history.

Defenses and distorted attributions. Those who have worked with child abusers, rapists, and other sexual abusers will be aware of the significant extent to which the offender has developed and skillfully utilizes an elaborate set of rationalizations. Rapists, for example, may claim that the victim "wanted it," "enjoyed it," "needed it," and "deserved it." The rationalizations employed by offending clinicians can be similar. They claim that the patient was seductive, that the patient would benefit only by erotic contact, or that the patient "consented." The damage that therapist-patient contact causes is minimized and discounted if not denied altogether. The patient's sexual history, sexual orientation, or sexual desires are brought up to justify the therapist's actions. Each of these possible defenses and attributions needs to be carefully explored and worked through.

Honesty and openness. Sexual exploitation of a patient is a serious offense. It is something that future employers, patients, and others deserve to be aware of. Knowing that a therapist has sexually exploited a patient might be crucially important to a parent who is selecting a child therapist, to an incest victim looking for treatment, or to a victim of therapist-patient sex seeking a subsequent therapist. In such cases, consent to treatment can hardly be termed "informed" if it is based on ignorance of the therapist's sexual offense. If any of us were investing money, would we feel that we had a right to know whether our financial adviser had been convicted of fraud? A similar principle obtains here. Prospective patients and employers, for example, deserve to know about an instance of abuse as serious as therapist-patient sexual contact. To the extent that an offending therapist is unwilling to be open and honest about his or her history in this regard, the denial, defensiveness, and lack of forthrightness are continuing and rehabilitation cannot be said to be complete. [Note: Hospitals, clinics, and other institutions that employ therapists must, to avoid negligence, seek reliable information concerning whether prospective clinical employees have been found—by a licensing board, by a professional organization, or by the courts—to have engaged in sex with a patient.]

Resources for prevention. It is not just that the rehabilitation process must work through and eliminate the risk factors for sexual exploitation in therapists. Offending clinicians must develop extensive and reliable resources for coping with sudden or unanticipated risks and temptations that may occur in the future. Methods for developing such resources are discussed by Pope (1987).

CONCLUSION

The days of the "old boy" self-protective network with its conspiracy of silence (in which professionals refused to express negative opinions about even the most outrageous behavior of their colleagues, let alone testify that the behavior violated the accepted standard of care) are, mercifully, finally beginning to come to an end. More and more, those responsible for protecting the welfare of the consumer and for ensuring high professional standards are failing to accept superficial and pro forma rehabilitation efforts. Conducting rehabilitation efforts and assessing offending clinicians are no less important, complex, or serious professional tasks than treating schizophrenia or assessing the presence of neuropsychological impairment. It may be that the elimination of bogus rehabilitation efforts and of the overly hasty granting of "rehabilitated" status to offending therapists will be facilitated by malpractice suits filed against those who are less than adequately professional, careful, thorough, and knowledgeable in assessing and rehabilitating offending therapists. Regardless of the circumstances, mental health professionals cannot in good conscience continue to enable offenders to practice in the absence of reasonably persuasive evidence of rehabilitation.

SECTION TWO

Chapter 11

Sexual Exploitation by Sex Therapists

Leslie R. Schover, Ph.D.

The ethical standards of sex therapists must be like the morals of Caesar's wife—above reproach. Those who treat sexual problems tread a thin line between expert assessment and voyeurism, prescribing behavior and intrusiveness. To practice sex therapy effectively, a clinician must develop clear boundaries between her or his own sexual needs and values and those of the patient.

Like incestuous fathers who justify their behavior by labeling it as "sex education," a number of psychotherapists seduce patients into sexual contact under the guise of "sex therapy" (Pope and Bouhoutsos 1986). I believe that sexual contact with patients is rarely reported, however, for therapists with specialized practices in behavioral sex therapy. This impression was reinforced in a discussion with Kenneth Pope, author of other chapters in this volume and former chairman of the American Psychological Association's Ethics Committee.

Nevertheless, the American public is confused about the role of the sex therapist. It is not unusual for patients to reject a referral to sex therapy because they believe it entails sexual behavior in the office. A brief overview of the development of sex therapy as a discipline illustrates how this confusion arose.

THE DEVELOPMENT OF SEX THERAPY:
HOW DIRECT IS DIRECT TREATMENT?

Before Masters and Johnson published *Human Sexual Inadequacy* in 1970, the typical psychotherapy for a sexual problem was psychodynamic, although behaviorists already were pioneering techniques such as systematic desensitization for sexual dysfunction (Leiblum and Pervin 1980). The unique components of sex therapy included treating the couple as a unit, prescribing homework exercises such as sensate focus, and concentrating on current sexual attitudes and communication rather than on early childhood development.

The direct treatment of sexual dysfunction arrived in the thick of the sexual revolution. Perhaps it is not surprising, then, that behavioral techniques were commingled with the least enduring trappings of the human potential movement. In San Francisco, a series of explicit sex education films was made using counterculture volunteers and sitar music in the background. Hartman and Fithian (1972) advocated the sexological examination, in which a therapist took an opposite-gender patient into an examination room and, in the spouse's presence, manually stimulated the patient's genitals to demonstrate the sexual response cycle. I recall in the late 1970s, listening to a woman attending a meeting of the American Association of Sex Educators, Counselors, and Therapists (AASECT) describe her clinic. She employed both male and female "sensual guides" who engaged in genital touching with patients, although actual penile-vaginal intercourse did not take place. The therapist often observed the exercise through a one-way mirror, albeit with the patient's consent.

Masters and Johnson (1976) have denounced sexual contact between therapist and patient as a form of rape that deserves criminal prosecution, but their own work was distorted to justify some of these marginal "sex therapies." Unlike Kinsey et al. (1948, 1953), who based their research on human sexuality largely on verbal interviews, Masters and Johnson observed men and women masturbating or having intercourse in laboratory conditions. Their pioneering helped to legitimize the ethical study of human sexual physiology (Masters and Johnson 1966). Some "sex therapists" saw these observational techniques as part of treatment, although Masters and Johnson drew a clear line between studying the sexual response and assessing sexuality for the purpose of treating a dysfunction. In the sex therapy format they devised, assessment was based on an extensive series of interviews. Patients performed the sexual exercises in private and then described the experience to the cotherapy team (Masters and Johnson 1970).

In fact, one purpose of using a male-female cotherapy duo was to prevent any trespassing across sexual boundaries with patients. Even erotic attractions between cotherapists were examined for possible detrimental effects on treatment (Golden and Golden 1976; Zentner and Pouyat 1978).

THE SEXUAL SURROGATE CONTROVERSY

As long as a patient came to Masters and Johnson with a cooperative sexual partner, sex therapy could proceed. Given that sex therapy was created as a couple treatment, however, a dilemma arose about how to help patients who had no partner. The solution was to use middle-class female volunteers as "sexual surrogates," partners who would engage in the sex therapy exercises with the patient, teaching him skills and self-confidence that hopefully would carry over into more conventional sexual relationships. After Masters and Johnson (1970) published their successful results using surrogates, a number of other therapists took up the practice. A national association of sexual surrogates also was founded. Whereas some surrogates worked in tandem with a sex therapist, many made independent agreements with patients becoming, in essence, both surrogate and therapist. Masters and Johnson used only female surrogates, but other therapists employed men as well, both gay and heterosexual.

By the early 1980s most sex therapists stopped working with sexual surrogates. Masters and Johnson ceased the practice because of legal problems as well as the tendency of the surrogates to get emotionally involved with the wealthy patients (LoPiccolo 1978). Masters himself (Redlich 1977) deplored the phenomenon of a surrogate deciding to be the therapist instead of remaining a sexual partner for the patient. The AASECT Code of Ethics (1979) allows therapists to employ surrogates, but only with adequate supervision, consent of spouses if the surrogate or patient is married, and attention to protecting the patient's dignity, welfare, and confidentiality, including eliciting informed consent about legal, social, and psychological risks to patient and surrogate partner.

The Berkeley Sex Therapy Group has developed an exemplary "body therapy" program, but their work is unique (Apfelbaum 1984). For many single men and women with sexual dysfunctions, treatment in a group format (Mills and Kilmann 1982) or using sex therapy exercises in self-stimulation with imagery techniques (Zilbergeld 1978) can provide a foundation for initiating a more successful sexual relationship.

The AIDS epidemic is also bound to curtail the surrogate movement. Not only would a sexual surrogate be at risk to contract the HIV because of having multiple sexual partners, but neither surrogate nor client could be guaranteed to be seronegative for HIV. It may take 4 months between exposure to the virus and development of a positive response to an antibody test (Goedert 1987). Although the potential partners could agree to submit to a sexual quarantine period, how could their compliance be verified?

SEXUAL BOUNDARIES IN SEX THERAPY

Sex therapy has often been touted as a simple type of treatment, well-suited to paraprofessionals. Yet, a competent sex therapist needs to be expert in individual, marital, and group therapy and to understand recent advances in medical assessment and treatment of sexual problems (Schover and Jensen 1988). A sex therapist should be, by my definition, a fully trained mental health professional, bound by the ethical constraints described in the rest of this volume. Codes of ethics have also been adopted by specialized professional societies such as AASECT or the Society for Sex Therapy and Research. These organizations agree that sex between patient and therapist is unethical.

Gray areas still exist. For example the AASECT Code of Ethics (1979) states that nudity or direct observation of sexual activity "may be used only when there is good evidence that they serve the best interests of the client." I do not believe that such evidence exists. Nudity or observation of sex can be emotionally intrusive and potentially harmful to a fragile patient (Pope and Bouhoutsos 1986).

Safe alternatives are also readily available. If a woman wants to become more comfortable with nudity, the therapist can assign her a graduated series of behavioral assignments to expose her body in a nonthreatening and appropriate way to her sexual partner. If a couple wants to observe the physiological changes of the male or female sexual response, the therapist can show them one of the excellent educational videotapes made for that purpose. Later the partners can observe each other's bodies in the privacy of their own home. A skilled interviewer can also derive a clear picture of the process of a sensate focus exercise by detailed questioning. Direct observation of a sexual interaction is not necessary. In fact, the variable of most interest is each partner's subjective experience of the interaction. The exact technique a husband used in caressing his wife's clitoris is not nearly as important as each partner's perception of how the wife guided his hand or gave him feedback.

For example, I recently treated a couple whose 6-year marriage had never been consummated because of the wife's severe vaginismus. When examined under anesthesia by a gynecologist, she was found to have a normal vagina and vulva. Therapy started out optimistically. Both partners learned about genital anatomy from life-like models. The wife looked at her genitals in the mirror at home, found the vaginal introitus, and learned to control her pubococcygeal muscles. She became stalled for several weeks, however, because she could use relaxation techniques to stay calm while she rested a finger on the vaginal opening, but could not bring herself to slide a finger into her vagina.

As she discussed her doubts that she had a normal vagina and her difficulty in finding the angle at which to insert a fingertip into the introitus, I was tempted to have her examine herself in my office, where I could coach her and help her maintain enough relaxation to try the next step. We came up with two alternatives, however, that did not have the potential for her misinterpreting my helpfulness as seduction or violation of her sexual boundaries. One was to have her husband hold her in his arms at home the next time she tried the exercise of inserting her finger into her vagina. He was very supportive, and she could allow him to check that she was touching the right place. Another option was for me to be present along with her female gynecologist in the gynecologist's office for an in vivo coaching session. The combination of these two techniques was successful in breaking the impasse. Although progress continued to be slow, the patient was learning that she had control over her own sexuality.

SOME FACTORS FAVORING SAFETY IN SEX THERAPY

I see sex therapists as less vulnerable to the temptation to act out sexually with patients for several reasons. One safety valve may be habituation. Even among health professionals, sex therapy is a titillating topic. It involves some of our most intense emotions. Medical students remember vivid aspects of their human sexuality courses such as watching explicit films or hearing a panel of gay men discuss their sexuality. Being a sex therapist, however, is like working for a while in an ice cream store. After you have sampled all the flavors, ice cream no longer makes your mouth water. I restrict my analogy to the voyeuristic aspects of sexuality. I do not believe that sex therapy detracts from the therapist's own sexual relationships. I am not often aroused, however, by hearing the details of someone else's sex life, unless the story evokes some image that taps into my own eroticism. Indeed, to me it is relationships and intimacy that are fascinating, not the multiplicity of intercourse positions, erogenous zones, or triggers for orgasm.

Another feature of competent sex therapy is that it empowers the patient, not the therapist. Like other behavior therapies, its goal is education through a series of success experiences. If sex therapists use self-disclosure, it is usually to model adaptive coping, rather than to illustrate sexual mastery. For example, a therapist might recall some myths about masturbation from his own adolescence or recount an awkward experience of first intercourse. Another aspect of empower-ment is that in working with a couple, the therapist is the outsider consulting with them on making their intimate communication work. This stance is antithetical to the intrusive, controlling position of a therapist who uses the transference relationship to seduce a patient.

A third characteristic of sex therapy that militates against sex between therapist and patient is the demystification of sexuality. For most of us, sexual attraction rests to some extent on novelty. We discover the unknown in our partners, mapping their bodies, their erotic preferences, their vulnerabilities. Love, and the complex thera-peutic relationship, can survive quite a bit of demystification. Motiva-tion and personality are endlessly fascinating. The sexually arousing aspects of novelty are much more fragile, however. After the clinician has heard about a woman's fears that her breasts are too small and that she has an unpleasant genital odor—when he knows the exact type of stimulation she uses during masturbation—becoming her sexual partner would not be a conquest or an exploration.

Patients almost invariably disclose more about their sexuality during a sex therapy assessment interview than they ever had with a partner. In fact, I think that engaging in sensate focus exercises and working on sexual communication often temporarily de-eroticize sex for patients during sex therapy. It is only when partners have gained enough knowledge about each other's technical needs that playful-ness, tenderness, and passion completely banish the mechanical feel-ing.

TRAINING THERAPISTS TO AVOID VOYEURISM AND COPE WITH ATTRACTION TO PATIENTS

Novice therapists need specific training to assess sexual problems and treat them effectively. Although part of the training is learning what questions to ask, how to design behavioral treatment programs, and how to debrief sex therapy homework, another crucial skill is managing one's own issues of voyeurism and attraction to patients.

Many clinicians feel flustered and incompetent in merely discussing the topic of sexuality with a patient. Therapists need to examine their own sexual values and minimize areas of discomfort. A sex therapist must be able to elicit the details of a patient's sexual practices and fantasies. These skills have rarely been studied in real-life sex therapy, but an analogue study suggested that male therapists with conservative sexual attitudes avoided focusing on a woman's complaint of orgasmic dysfunction. Female therapists or men with more liberal sexual attitudes responded to the analogue patient more therapeutically (Schover 1981).

Therapists may fear a patient's seductiveness. In a series of sex therapy training seminars for health professionals in Denmark, male therapists' most common anxiety about using their new skills was that they would feel attracted to a female patient. Women therapists, in contrast, feared a male patient would be angry or aggressively sexual (Jensen and Mohl 1987). Again in the analogue study just cited, if a therapist was confronted by a seductive patient, the male therapist–female patient pairing produced the most troublesome responses. Male therapists were more apt to avoid dealing with a female patient's sexual advances and judged the seductive patient more harshly (Schover 1981). Thus, men fear temptation from their own impulses, whereas women therapists can handle flirtation, but dread overt sexual aggression from the patient.

I do believe that male and female clinicians elicit different responses when discussing sex with opposite-gender patients. Although I am a female therapist dealing much of the time with male sexual dysfunctions, I rarely receive sexual propositions. One reason may be the power imbalance of the therapy relationship. In our society, male sexuality is synonymous with the one-up position. After spending a session describing his sexual failures and vulnerabilities, a man is unlikely to feel sexually attracted to the therapist. The dynamics are different for the male therapist–female patient dyad. It is easy for the female patient to feel drawn to the powerful therapist because power inequality parallels gender stereotypes.

If a male patient makes a sexual remark to me, it usually has a hostile undertone, for example, "Are you sure you wouldn't be a sex surrogate for me?" or "What's your sex life like?" The message is resentment of my professional role. I try to use these interactions as a stimulus for discussing the pressures on men to be "sex experts" and as an example of the pain and anger the patient may feel in acknowledging his own vulnerability.

Maladaptive therapist responses to patients' sexual issues can arise from faulty beliefs. Each clinician should carefully examine and challenge these attitudes during training and clinical supervision.

Faulty Belief 1: A competent therapist should never feel sexually aroused during a session. Patients evoke the whole range of emotions in therapists. The skill of therapy does not rest in being unfeeling, but rather in recognizing one's own emotions and untangling their sources. Sex therapy, in particular, entails discussing erotic activities. If a therapist is sexually aroused because a patient's description of sex evokes a pleasant memory, the arousal is probably irrelevant to the therapy process. Refocusing on the patient is in order. If the therapist is aroused because an attractive male patient is making intense eye contact and sitting in a way that reveals he has an erection, the sexual feeling is part of the interaction. The therapist should consider whether a discussion of the sexual signals would be therapeutic. Perhaps the patient often uses seductiveness to get attention and nurturance from women, but then is upset when women want intimacy. The therapy relationship illustrates this pattern and given the understanding that no sexual contact is going to take place, provides a safe context to explore it.

As Searles (1959) has pointed out, the therapist's arousal may indicate that the patient has become more sexually attractive as he or she has resolved some psychopathology and can relate to the therapist in a more mature way. I find in sex therapy that I am rarely aroused by a patient recounting a scene of sexual disaster, but I may feel aroused at the end of treatment when a couple describes a pleasurable sexual interaction that was playful or tender, and free from crippling anxiety.

Training should include role-playing scenarios of becoming aroused with a patient while discussing sexual material. The supervisor can provide suggestions on how to respond appropriately.

Faulty Belief 2: If I am attracted to a patient, I am in danger of acting out sexually. Our society indoctrinates teenagers that sexual arousal is an uncontrollable passion. Excitement leads to kissing, petting, and ultimately intercourse. President Carter "confesses" to lusting in his heart, and it is only his strong religious beliefs that prevent adultery. Young men try to coax women into sexual activity by invoking "blue balls," claiming that severe pain and possibly permanent testicular damage will result from frustrated desire.

It is not surprising, then, that therapists fear a sexual attraction to a patient will get out of control. Sex becomes a topic that is best avoided. Yet, sexual arousal is no more frightening or dangerous than other strong emotions that therapists experience and learn to manage, such as anger, guilt, or the wish to "rescue" the patient.

Therapists are less afraid of their sexual feelings when they have clear boundaries about intimate contacts with patients. If a clinician knows that he or she limits touching with patients to a hug or handshake, the discussion in session can focus on sexual impulses or feelings. There is no need to debate whether sexual contact should take place. As illustrated by the survey research of Pope et al. (1986), the great majority of therapists feel attracted to patients occasionally.

A sex therapist who feels strongly attracted to a patient has a number of choices. If sex therapy is conducted by a cotherapy team, the therapist should discuss the issue openly with his or her colleague. When cotherapists respect and like each other, as they must to work effectively, they need to share their emotional reactions to the patient couple. The cotherapist can help his or her partner figure out why the attraction is occurring and monitor its impact during the therapy session.

More commonly sex therapists work alone, since cotherapy is uneconomical and is not necessary for effective sex therapy (Arentewicz and Schmidt 1983; LoPiccolo et al. 1985). In that situation, the best way to manage a sexual attraction to a patient is to seek supervision by a colleague. The focus of supervision should be on the source of the attraction (patient behavior, therapist's history, etc.), whether the therapist should disclose to the patient any observations about the attraction (i.e., if it reflects the patient's typical style of interaction with others or is disrupting the therapy process), and how to resolve the strong emotions in the most therapeutic way for the patient. Occasionally, referral to another therapist may be necessary.

Faulty Belief 3: *I am an expert in sexuality and could cure my patients with my skilled lovemaking.* Although no legitimate sex therapist has advocated therapist-patient sexual contact, some clinicians have extrapolated from the use of sexual surrogates and the direct behavioral assignments given in sex therapy a belief that they could cure sexual dysfunctions by personal sexual intervention. In the survey of 1,423 members of the American Psychiatric Association described in Chapter 1, 4.5 percent felt therapist-patient contact could be helpful in treating sexual dysfunction. Although many of these respondents specified the contact would be with a surrogate rather than the therapist himself or herself, 18 percent of 84 therapists who admitted to having sex with patients saw it as an appropriate intervention for sexual dysfunction. Seven percent of the acting-out group believed therapist-patient sex could change a patient's sexual orientation. The grandiosity of such attitudes hardly needs comment, except to note that therapists who have sex with patients are often intrusive in other ways, setting themselves up as arbiters of every aspect of their patients' lives (Pope and Bouhoutsos 1986).

FUTURE DIRECTIONS

To prevent sexual abuse of patients in the name of "sex therapy," improvements are needed in training and in licensure laws. All psychotherapists, whether psychologists, psychiatrists, or social workers, need training in assessing and treating sexual problems. Only the state of California has a requirement for training in sexuality for licensure of mental health professionals (Pope and Bouhoutsos 1986). Other states need to follow that lead. Training programs must also reexamine their curricula. A better understanding not only of ethical issues, but also of the techniques effective in treating sexual dysfunction, should prevent sexual exploitation of patients. These components of education cannot be presented adequately in one weekend workshop. Ideally a semester of course work plus supervision of several sex therapy cases should take place (Schover and Jensen 1988). Curriculum planners often regard sexuality as a frivolous topic, ignoring it or relegating it to an elective course. Yet, how many psychotherapies fail to at least touch on sexual issues? Masters and Johnson (1970) estimated that one-half of American couples have a sexual dysfunction at some point in their relationships. Subsequent surveys confirm that sexual problems are common even for young, healthy people and are ubiquitous in patients with chronic illnesses (Schover and Jensen 1988).

The day of seeing "sex therapy" as a bag of tricks that can be learned by a layperson is over. I strongly believe that states should restrict the title "sex therapist" and the practice of sex therapy under the same laws that govern generic psychotherapy. I also do not advocate peer support groups without a trained professional as a leader, for example for preorgasmic women or to discuss issues of gay sexuality. The potential not only for perpetuating misinformation, but for sexual victimization or coercion of group members is too high. In sex therapy treatment groups for patients without committed partners, the therapist should agree with all group members that no sexual contact will take place between them for the duration of the therapy. Most such groups are composed of same-gender heterosexual patients, which minimizes such risks.

In summary, I believe that training for every mental health clinician should include sensitization to the negative consequences of sex with patients, role playing and supervision on dealing with attraction to patients, and at least a basic course in the effective assessment and treatment of sexual problems. Only by attending to these issues will we prevent the sexual exploitation of patients in general, and stop sexual abuse perpetrated in the guise of sex therapy.

Chapter 12

Sexual Involvement Between Psychiatric Hospital Staff and Their Patients

Dean T. Collins, M.D.

Any informal, relaxed, and nondefensive discussion with administratively responsible personnel of a psychiatric hospital (e.g., administrator, medical director, or director of nursing) will elicit the fact that unethical relationships between staff members and patients constitute a significant personnel problem. Nonetheless, searches of the psychiatric literature on the subject reveal an astounding paucity of articles. Indeed, despite a growing volume of literature on sexual exploitation of patients, the references are almost exclusively to sexual exploitation by psychotherapists. Only two articles (Collins et al. 1978; Stone 1975) make specific reference to other hospital personnel.

While Stone's (1975) five cases refer to psychiatric residents in four instances, in the fifth both a male attendant and a male activities counselor are implicated. The attendant became sexually involved with a female patient. Several encounters had occurred within the hospital, all shortly before the vacation of the patient's therapist. The patient had been a close friend of another patient, who had committed suicide in the aftermath of an affair with her activities counselor. Stone highlights the need to reemphasize the functional aspects of the medical-psychiatric canons of professional comportment.

Collins et al. (1978) examined the impact of sexual contact with treaters on subsequent psychiatric treatment. A cohort of 15 patients reporting direct genital contact with a psychotherapist was contrasted with a comparison group of 18 patients reporting sexual contact with a staff member directly involved with their treatment, but in a role other than psychotherapist. They concluded that both groups experienced significant complications in subsequent treatment efforts. However, sexual activity with other treatment personnel may be viewed as a displacement of (and alternative to) the fantasied sexual contact with the psychotherapist, so its deleterious effects on later treatment are milder (but still significant) than sex directly with the therapist (the primary object of transference). Hospital treatment of the second group was dramatically characterized by issues of control between patient and treatment staff. Indeed, the sexual activity with one of the treatment staff could be viewed as the demonstration of the patient's ultimate "control" over the hospital staff.

As participants in, or managers of, hospital settings that provide a locus for treatment efforts aimed at assisting the patient in psychological change, we must all be aware that each of us is exposed to the occupational hazard of complications in our relationships with patients. The very tools we are using to accomplish change may be exploited: Social relationships may be pursued for a staff member's pleasure; financial relationships may be entered into for a staff member's gain; and romantic relationships may evolve that have the potential for sexual exploitation of the patient. There are many examples of practitioners whose intent was never to take advantage of the patient, but who were drawn insidiously into an eroticized interaction by the very intimacy that characterizes a therapeutic relationship.

When the staff members of a hospital are invited to discuss the occupational hazards of staff-patient relationships, their first thoughts are of physical contact—that is, assaultive, violent behavior or sexual relationships. But the hazards of staff-patient relationships include a wide spectrum of issues of which these behaviors are the extremes. Along this spectrum lie a number of disturbances in staff-patient relationships that serve as early warning signals. These should be evident by various clues that are sometimes subtle, sometimes so ubiquitous that they go unnoticed, unchecked, and often ignored. Nevertheless, when a problem becomes known, when something finally goes wrong, there is always someone around to say, "I could have told you so."

A night nursing supervisor received a phone message for one of the regular male staff members on the night shift. The supervisor knew that the staff member, when making rounds, frequently stopped to talk with a young female patient who always went to sleep late. On approaching that patient's room to give the staff member his message, the supervisor came to a disquieting realization. The door to the patient's room was closed. She knocked, then waited a few minutes for a response before finally opening the door, even though she fully expected the male staff member to be there. In retrospect, during a sexual misconduct investigation, she acknowledged that her hesitation at the door reflected her suspicion that sexual activity might be occurring behind the closed door. She regretted not sharing her suspicion with her supervisor.

APPROPRIATE STAFF-PATIENT RELATIONSHIPS

The central importance of staff-patient relationships in psychiatric hospital treatment is underscored by the emphasis on their various aspects during training, education, consultation, and research. This focus on the staff-patient relationship may result in discussions of the therapeutic or treatment alliance, transference and countertransference phenomena, ethics, and malpractice litigation. Such an emphasis is understandable, because much of a patient's response to psychiatric intervention, either psychological or biological, is dependent on and influenced by the nature of staff-patient relationships (e.g., motivation for treatment, treatment compliance, the placebo effect, and the power of suggestion).

We who work in treatment settings in which interpersonal relationships are considered to be among the forces for change must acknowledge the potential such relationships have for abuse or exploitation. Treatment settings that offer extended treatment for patients with borderline personality disorders or higher-level psychotic disorders may be particularly vulnerable. Paradoxically, the very relationships that offer the promise of healing to users of long-term psychiatric services also expose practitioners of all disciplines to the hazards of overstepping their professional bounds.

By emphasizing interpersonal relationships as major vehicles for helping, as well as by openly espousing the concept that all staff members in a hospital are active agents in the treatment process, we undeniably increase staff involvement, morale, and competence. However, difficulties arise when a staff member's wish to be helpful or to relate to a patient as a "friend" instead of as a "treatment figure" spurs that staff member into a relationship that is not part of the planned and supervised program. Also, depending on the size of the psychiatric hospital and its degree of integration into the surrounding community, there may be opportunities for many patients to encounter staff members in college classes, restaurants, taverns, movies, parties, and elsewhere. Thus our emphasis on the importance of relationships as vehicles for positive influence must also make us mindful of how relationships may impede or be antagonistic to treatment goals. Guidelines cannot cover every eventuality—but they should serve to stimulate thoughtful reflection on past, present, and future interactions with patients. In the final analysis, there is no substitute for the exercise of good judgment on the part of every staff member.

> A male social worker took his car for repairs at a local garage. He appeared to pick it up prior to coming to work, having allowed just enough time to make it to a team meeting. When he got to the garage, there was a female patient from his unit team who needed a ride (one who was also expected at the same team meeting). The mechanic, knowing that the woman was from the hospital, had informed her that someone else from the hospital, with whom she could catch a ride, would soon be there. The patient had agreed to wait. The social worker knew from staff discussions that the patient had many erotic fantasies about him. He was also aware that staff members were not to provide rides for patients in their personal cars. This policy immediately entered his mind—along with the thought that this was harmless, and nothing more than he would do for any other person. He drove her back to the hospital, and they both attended the team meeting.

This vignette illustrates how boundary violations may begin as simple acts of kindness or courtesy. Departing from established policy can always be rationalized under the guise of flexibility and humane concern for the patient.

A patient, of course, may regard some team members as wiser than others, some as more compassionate, and some as more likely to be of help. Correspondingly, team members sometimes regard themselves as having an especially good relationship with a patient or as understanding the patient better than others do. While some or all of these attitudes may actually be correct at any given time, patients tend to re-create in the hospital milieu the poorly integrated, primitive object relations that characterized their lives before admission. A complete understanding of the patient's object world can occur only by surveying the entire array of relationships. Thus, failures to deal with covert disagreements and splits within teams may perpetuate, if not intensify, intrapsychic conflicts (Stanton and Schwartz 1954). There is no question that a secret or clandestine relationship between a patient and one member of the treatment team signals a serious problem that may interfere with understanding and treating the patient.

The significance of a relationship between a patient and a staff member who is not directly connected with the patient's treatment is often less clear with respect to its possible pathologic origins and its influence on the treatment process. Such relationships may be purely social, neither intended to help nor to be influenced by the ongoing treatment process. The key issue is whether such relationships can truly be unmotivated by or unaffected by factors related to a patient's treatment. All staff members of a psychiatric hospital are ultimately most helpful to patients if their relationships exist within a team-monitored treatment plan. The character of those relationships must therefore be accessible to the treatment team for review and supervision. To help prevent inappropriate interactions with patients, staff members must first be aware of how such relationships might develop and then must be open to discussing the resolution of such problem relationships.

Transference does not respect team or section boundaries, and the motivations for a relationship between a patient and a staff member may be exceedingly complex for each party. Although many patients are interesting people with a wealth of experiences and abilities in addition to their difficulties, the disadvantages to the patient in these relationships appear to outweigh the advantages. The difficulty in understanding what such a relationship ultimately means to a patient, and what impact it has on the treatment, suggests a cautious attitude toward developing such relationships. Almost by definition, a large number of mental hospital patients cannot define nor constructively manage their interpersonal relationships, unlike better functioning outpatients, who may be able to explore all relationships systematically within psychotherapy.

AVOIDING INAPPROPRIATE RELATIONSHIPS

To avoid "initiating" friendships—that is, making repetitive social contacts with the aim of mutual enjoyment—by no means implies that staff members must be unfriendly to patients. However, offering or responding to an overture for some social, recreational, or romantic involvement carries the risk of participating in splitting or transference-countertransference acting out that might ultimately be detrimental to the patient.

It is certainly true that many patients are lonely and socially inept, and so staff members may wish to offer friendship as a way of facilitating social learning and rehabilitation. However, the hospital should not be seen as a place where patients come to find friendship, but rather as a setting where they can develop the capacity for relating to others so that capacity can be used for establishing independent relationships. Treatment figures should be transitional figures in that a treatment relationship should be a means to the end of enhanced abilities to deal with others, not a specifically provided substitute that is an end in itself.

In turn, staff members should not have to use patients as resources for friendships. They should have independently satisfying personal lives so as not to be dependent on patients for their social pleasures. In addition, staff members should always help patients define their mutual roles in terms of the treatment contract and should not offer more or less than is reasonable within that contract.

PROFILE OF THE VULNERABLE PATIENT

In reviewing numerous instances of staff-patient sexual relationships in private, state, and federal hospitals, the following profile emerges:

1. The history of the patient vulnerable to sexual exploitation by a staff member may include any of the following: incest or other sexual abuse in childhood; previous sexual exploitation by teachers, counselors, or therapists (in childhood or young adult years); a lack of memory for extended periods during childhood; or more general interpersonal boundary violations or physical abuse by caretakers.
2. The vulnerable patient is often characterized by some features of borderline personality disorder, particularly splitting (into good and bad treaters, with "special" staff members); treatment resistance or defeating mechanisms; the evoking of rescue fantasies in staff members; a tendency to keep secrets out of mistrust; and a fear of revenge (especially by being dismissed from treatment).
3. The patient is often conscious of a desire to be reassured that he or she is liked, found attractive, cared for, or nurtured. There may

also be a wish to be touched, hugged, or held for comfort, and a wish to be cuddled as a major component of sexual activity.

4. When the patient is female (as is usually the case), there may be a subtle anger toward a significant male figure. This may stem from interactions with a father who was either overinvolved in a "special relationship" or neglectful. Subsequent relationships with males may have hinted at a struggle for power, wherein the "secret" aspect of the relationship that transgresses usual staff-patient boundaries, or is overtly sexual, bonds the powerful male to her. This shared secret thus assures continuity of the relationship.

5. The themes in the treatment of the vulnerable patient often include: issues of control, revenge, or sadism; difficulties with separations and losses (accompanied by acting out); interpersonal boundary violations; complaints of injustices; secretiveness and a relationship with treating staff that may give the appearance of a therapeutic alliance, but actually may be deceptive and misleading—a pseudotherapeutic alliance.

6. Conditions that have been associated with sexual exploitation often include dissociative states, multiple personality, and anorgasmia (particularly selective, e.g., with the spouse only).

In summary, the typical patients are those with borderline personality disorders who have complained of "emptiness" and have displaced object hunger with a propensity to seek out affect-intensifying experiences. They are seen as treatment resistant and/or actively treatment defeating. They have a history of childhood sexual abuse or a history that suggests it. They are people who have made staff angry with them and have pushed staff away in many different ways. They are generally seen as not improving in treatment. They are typically involved in an extended treatment process where opportunities for transference may be maximal. Despite staff difficulties in trusting them, however, they are able to evoke sympathy and to invite one staff member to help them. To this privileged treater they have indicated that he or she is special and can provide what others cannot (Gabbard 1986, E. Zoble, personal communication, April 3, 1986).

PROFILE OF THE STAFF MEMBER VULNERABLE TO SEXUAL EXPLOITATION OF A PATIENT

Vulnerable staff were of both sexes, all ages, and of no particular socioeconomic background. [It should be recognized that more direct psychological data are generally available on patients than on staff members—descriptions of the latter are based on administrative and supervisory observations.] There were, however, two general categories. One category was the new staff member, who passed through a screening process without recognition of his or her history of being sexually exploitative, and who continued to carry on that exploitation in the psychiatric hospital setting with relatively vulnerable people. The other category was the middle-aged person, isolated and alone, having some significant difficulties in his or her personal life and a need for nurture.

With the first category, the sexually exploitative staff member responds to the patient's narcissistic strivings, recognizing and identifying with the patient's own wishes to be special. Simultaneously, there may be an unconscious wish to have the patient act out and successfully usurp authority vis-à-vis the organization.

The staff member in the second category is susceptible to entering into an exclusive, idealized position that invites secretiveness. He or she then rationalizes this clandestine behavior because it is ego-syntonic. The intense nature of this dyad taps into that particular staff member's unconscious desire to be better and/or more special than others, thus the ultimate caregiver. The process is mutually seductive—the patient attempts to be special to the staff member, while the staff member, in turn, is more vulnerable to yielding to his or her own desire to retain the specialness of that relationship.

The difficulties of a patient described in the above patient profile may tend to appeal to staff narcissism and to rescue fantasies. A person undergoing a crisis in his or her personal life may be especially susceptible to this development. Vulnerable staff members may be those who feel sexually conflicted and dissatisfied, who themselves are angry with the institution, and who feel that they have been wronged by it. They may feel that their efforts at recognition have been thwarted. They may be people who are performers or who have exhibitionistic features. If staff members have all these features, they seem to be vulnerable to explicit or implied seductiveness and may collude with a patient to maintain secrecy about their relationship. Sexual exchanges may or may not be involved.

When the staff member has overstepped the boundaries (or the relationship has become too intense), the patient is more likely to disclose the nature of the relationship, and thus attempt to destroy and to devour the staff member. The latter defends against this development, possibly because it matches an aggressive, exploitative aspect of his or her own motivation. Following this outcome, the staff member may feel betrayed and may be unable to accept any responsibility for the relationship. The staff members are often married, respected professionals who are seen by peers as possessing integrity. When exposed, they are often crushed and cannot understand why the hospital administrator is not more sympathetic to their situation—an attitude that reflects a profound denial of social reality. Many of them are shocked when asked to leave employment, having rationalized or used other defenses to make their transgressions acceptable to themselves (E. Zoble, personal communication, April 3, 1986).

PREVENTION

Several resources within the psychiatric hospital can help staff members prevent or minimize the antitherapeutic hazards of relationships with patients. Such resources include clear policies and guidelines for all staff members, the use of consultation with colleagues and senior clinicians, and careful supervision—individual and group, clinical and administrative. We have also found it useful to utilize staff meetings or inservice training sessions as a forum in which to hold discussions of the occupational hazards involved in staff-patient relationships by presenting a staff group with vignettes designed to elicit reactions to specific situations.

Vignette 1. Ms. X has been working out and playing racquetball at a local racquet club for several years. It is not uncommon for a number of the members to go out for drinks or to get together in small groups for other activities. A few current and discharged patients have always used the facility. In the past year their numbers have increased. Ms. X knows most of them and has worked directly with some. Recently, one has been persistent in trying to "team up" with her for racquetball, which she has so far avoided with some flimsy excuse. Now she is finding it harder and harder to turn down his request. This person has started joining the group at a local bar after workouts on Monday evenings. Ms. X believes that she's in a dilemma: She does not want to give up her valued activity; however, she fears that if this situation continues, there will be problems with the patient. What should she do in this situation?
- Continue frequenting the racquet club?
- Avoid the patient like the plague but continue her activities?

- Continue her activities and proceed as usual?
- Talk to her supervisor about the dilemma?
- Suppose she does talk to her supervisor. How should the supervisor respond?

Vignette 2.   The team social worker has a very good relationship with the parents of a hospitalized patient. They congratulate her warmly on learning of her upcoming marriage and bring a beautifully wrapped gift to her at the time of the last session before her vacation. She returns the gift without opening it, explaining that clinical experience shows that gift-giving tends to complicate treatment relationships. The parents, obviously hurt, are polite, distant, and guarded in their subsequent dealings with the hospital staff. What could have made for a different outcome in this situation?

Vignette 3.   An eloped patient is located during a search but refuses to return to the hospital unless a particular staff member, who has not had the required defensive driving course, will drive her in his personal vehicle. Staff know from experience that the patient will put up a physical struggle if frustrated, possibly leading to law enforcement involvement and resulting commitment proceedings. It is only a few blocks back to the hospital. What should the staff member do?

Vignette 4.   Mr. J is your barber and a relatively good friend of yours. Over the years, you have shared a lot, visiting each other and having long discussions about your personal lives. You are aware that Mr. J is sometimes moody but so are most people. You are distressed by the news from his wife that he has made a suicide attempt and is now admitted to the crisis unit of the hospital where you work. Thinking this admission will be short-lived, and wanting to protect confidentiality, you decide not to visit him, to stop eating in the dining room, and to avoid going to that unit. You tell no one that you know Mr. J Returning to work after 2 days off, you learn that Mr. J is being transferred to the extended treatment unit on which you work. You can no longer avoid your friend. What are you to do? Should you have informed your supervisor earlier? At this point, how will you handle the situation?

Vignette 5.   A hospital social worker is counseling a patient and his wife in intense marital work revolving around the couple's sexual relationship. As the patient's discharge draws near, the wife plans to move closer to the hospital so that they can continue the marital work on an outpatient basis. In one of the sessions, the couple announce that they have made a down payment and signed a contract on a home, which the social worker realizes is next door to her home. What should she do?

Vignette 6. A patient with a history of abuse and rejection at the hand of a psychotic mother forms a strong attachment to a female nurse and unexpectedly presents her with a crystal pendant at Christmas. The accompanying card reads, "I know you won't refuse this the way my mother refused all my gifts." What should the nurse do?

Vignette 7. Everyone is in agreement with the plan for the team social worker to make a home visit with the patient to the patient's extended family in the western plains. The nearest hotel is 100 miles away and the patient's parents are insistent that the social worker stay in their spacious ranch home. To drive back and forth will increase the length and expense of the home visit. What should the social worker do?

Vignette 8. You enter a restaurant with several friends not associated with the hospital and are seated at a table immediately adjacent to where a patient and her husband are sitting with their teenaged children, whom you have not yet met. The patient and husband bring the teenagers to your table and start a round of introductions, extending handshakes to your friends and waiting to be introduced. How would you handle this situation?

General guidelines. Discussion of the foregoing vignettes serves a useful function in the education of hospital staff members. They promote an awareness of the ever-present potential for boundary violations and prepare treaters for situations in which they might otherwise have been caught off guard.

The following aphorisms have been found to be useful. They certainly are not all-encompassing, nor are they intended to be rules for conduct; rather, they are intended to illustrate a philosophy that each clinician must forge for himself or herself in the course of a career of helping disturbed people.

1. If a policy governing staff-patient relationships must be quoted by a staff member to strengthen his or her position, then that staff member's countertransference should be discussed in supervision.

2. Selective sharing of a staff member's own life experiences may be useful to a patient in certain circumstances, but such anecdotes should come from the staff member's past experience rather than from current problems or events.
3. Any development in a relationship with a patient that seems as if it should stay secret should be discussed in detail with one's supervisors or co-workers.
4. The knowledge one gains as a treater can never be erased as a potential influence in any subsequent relationship with a former patient.
5. The gratification and source of reward from one's work should, for the most part, derive from co-workers and colleagues. When they derive predominantly from patient relationships, the risk of problems and countertransference manifestations increases.
6. Once having accepted the role of treater for another person, one is never again as free as the person being treated. Even after termination of treatment, the former treater remains constrained by special knowledge of the circumstances. Therefore the former patient must have the freedom to choose no subsequent contact, even years later. The former treater is constrained to avoid any pursuit of social contacts.

SUMMARY

Because interpersonal relationships are significant forces in psychiatric treatment, we must be alert to the occupational hazard of overinvolvement for all who work with patients, especially those in hospital settings. Supervisors and managers must be alert to indicators that staff members are vulnerable to transgressing the boundaries of professional and therapeutic relationships with patients. Their responsibility is to utilize all the resources available to them to protect the patient, the process of treatment, and the professions.

Chapter 13

Teacher-Student Sexual Intimacy

Kenneth S. Pope, Ph.D.

The other chapters in this volume suggest that therapist-patient sex has received far too little attention from the profession. But if therapist-patient sex is something we have neglected, teacher-student sex is something we hardly acknowledge. Even our most probing texts tend to be silent on the subject. The eyes of those entrusted with our training programs are discreetly averted. It is a phenomenon which, on the professional level, is not seen, is not heard, and is not discussed. It is, of course, done quite frequently. It just can't be acknowledged and discussed as a professional concern. It remains the stuff of juicy gossip among students and, usually separately, among faculty, the underground tales of who is doing it with whom, who is "good" or "easy," what certain individuals have already gotten or can expect in return, and so on.

THE BASIC SCENARIOS

Just as most—but by no means all—instances of therapist-patient sexual involvement fall into 10 basic categories (Pope and Bouhoutsos 1986), most—but again not all—instances of educator-student sexual involvement seem to cluster into distinct groups, each with its own dynamics and course of development. The following 7 are typical.

Aladdin's Lamp. The student views the educator as the source of rare treasures. What does the student desire? An extremely high grade, perhaps. A sterling letter of recommendation to a highly competitive job, the type of letter that begins, "Not since Freud. . . ." Financial support for next year's studies. Mentorship and the accompanying entree into the rarefied atmosphere of the "truly important" in the field. In some cases, simply the undivided, favorable attention of the teacher seems to fill the heart with joy.

If the student truly desires such a treasure, and sees the professor, supervisor, or administrator as the source, what does the student need to do? As in the ancient myths and enchantment tales, there's a catch. Quite a catch.

The Offer That Can't Be Refused. Where rewards are ineffective or simply not available, threats of dire consequences are sometimes used to shape behavior. Nothing explicit, of course. To my knowledge, no educator has yet prepared a contract to be signed, notarized, and filed with the authorities along the lines of,

> I [student's name], will engage in sex with my professor in private and on a weekly basis. I realize that if I fail to meet the terms of this contract, I may invite consequences which may include but are not limited to the following: (1) the phase of my professor's research project on which I am working will be quickly completed, my services will no longer be needed, and I will lose my weekly check for those services; (2) the professor will give me a failing grade in his course; and (3) the professor will sadly, reluctantly, be forced to voice his concern about me in a confidential faculty meeting, pointing out how my behavior meets the DSM-III-R criteria for borderline personality disorder, acknowledging that his attempts to counsel me to mend my ways have been futile, and suggesting—though it is with the greatest disappointment that he finds himself forced to this conclusion—that, as the faculty member who best knows me and my work, he believes that I should be terminated from the training program and urged to consider other lines of work.

Students quickly learn the ropes, and educators can be quite adept at making clear, through indirection, what's expected (i.e., required).

Don Juan. This educator is a party animal—a swinger. The training institution is, to this professional, like a private game reserve or a well-stocked lake, replenished every year. Emotional entangle-ments are avoided, at least by the predator. An occasional student, of course, may unwittingly (and wrongly) assume that the sexual adven-ture entails some lasting emotional ties. Such false assumptions are firmly attributed to the student's immaturity, emotional "hang-ups," and possible thought disorder.

The Fountain of Youth.   Many of the educators in this category are in the throes of midlife or later-life crisis. In any event, they tend to experience their world as dry and constricted. Teaching is not much fun anymore, and they haven't revised their lecture notes in at least 5 years. They rarely know the names of all the students in their class. They wish that their offices were clean, well-lit places, but the hallmark is clutter. The main thing they await with genuine eagerness is for the end of the day's class, which seems never to come. Lines from Eliot and Beckett run through their thoughts. They wonder if they should have gone into another line of work. If they are single, they regret never marrying. If they are married, they regret not having remained single. If they are divorced, they regret everything.

Without warning, that special student jumps into their lives: young, beautiful in the eyes of the beholder, full of life and enthusi-asm and energy of every kind, including sexual. Who could say no to such a gift? Who could resist giving (or being) such a gift?

These relationships, while almost never "one-night stands," tend to run a relatively short course. The dynamics are often similar to what Weiner (1980) terms the "most common pathological love rela-tionship in our culture: the wedding of the hysteric with the obses-sive" (p. 128).

The obsessive . . . looks like a good parent to the hysteric. The hysteric is a welcome relief to the obsessive's permanently gray world. One's soberness and the other's cheerfulness should complement each other nicely. As it becomes apparent that the obsessive is more of a prison warden than a stabilizer for the hysteric, and that the hysteric's cheer-fulness lasts only as long as he or she is indulged, one of the partners becomes symptomatic. The hysteric becomes depressed or develops emotionally based physical symptoms. The compulsive becomes angry, feels persecuted, becomes more rigidly self-righteous, or becomes sus-picious of his or her mate's fidelity, as the mate flirts with others to feign independence and to maintain the endless stream of attention necessary to feed his or her self-esteem. (Weiner 1980, p. 128)

Frozen Roles. Similar in some ways to the "Fountain of Youth" pairing, "Frozen Roles" involves two individuals who seek an emotional/sexual/romantic relationship that embodies, preserves, and expresses the imbalance of authority, power, status, etc., which characterizes the formal and professional relationship between professor (or supervisor, administrator, etc.) and student. Neither educator nor student has been genuinely successful at maintaining an intimate relationship with a true equal, someone who does not chronically occupy a superior or subordinate, a dominant or dependent, role. The student always has someone to look up to (figuratively, at least). Because the individuals are so comfortable with the power and status differential, this pairing is the one most likely to be preserved for years and to result in marriage.

Before I Knew What Was Happening ...   Under the best and worst of circumstances, learning tends to be an emotionally charged experience. The laboratory and field research conducted by a variety of social psychologists indicates that interpersonal attraction—if only temporary—tends to be evoked or facilitated under such conditions of emotional arousal.

The interpersonal attraction that occurs in formal learning relationships may be fostered not only by the general emotional excitement but also by specific aspects of education. Therapists learn—or at least should learn—early in their training that patients are likely to experience transference as part of the therapy, and that many patients may "fall in love with" their therapists. Freud (1915) and subsequent therapists caution that therapists should not flatter themselves that such attraction is the same phenomenon that occurs outside the therapeutic situation. Therapists must recognize the transference phenomenon for what it is, respect it, and not exploit it.

Similarly, a kind of transference is prone to occur between student and teacher. Recognition of this phenomenon goes back at least to the ancient Greeks. Plato's (1967) account of Socrates, in discussing the ideas of Diotima, stresses the tendency of students to invest the teacher with the exciting, desirable, and fulfilling qualities associated with knowledge itself and the content being taught.

Some teachers may, like some therapists, exploit this phenomenon. The intimacy and excitement of education, and the resulting vulnerability of the student, are not sufficiently respected nor professionally handled by these professors. As they frequently describe it, they become lost in the intensity of the pedagogic relationship and gradually or suddenly, "before I knew what was happening," the teacher-student relationship becomes sexualized.

The Objective and Fair-Minded Educator. Some educators claim powers of objectivity and fair-mindedness that set them apart from their teaching colleagues, who are merely human. These educators can sleep one night a week with one of the students in a class and not let that intimate activity influence in any way the assigning of final grades. They can share an apartment with a student in a training program and have it not affect their judgment one bit when it comes to assigning fellowships and teaching assistantships. They can resonate with the passion of "true love" and a wonderfully fulfilling sex life with a student and retain their objectivity intact when they lend the authority, prestige, and integrity of their name to an enthusiastic and detailed letter recommending their lover for a job as a therapist at a hospital (so certain are they that the love affair is not affecting their judgment that they omit mention of it from the letter).

RESEARCH FINDINGS

There are four national studies yielding data about sexual intimacies between mental health educators (teachers, supervisors, and administrators) and their students, all in the field of psychology. We have no compelling reason to believe that the essential findings would be significantly different in psychiatry, social work, marriage counseling, or other disciplines, but we are in need of comparable national studies for those professions.

The initial study examined anonymous responses from 481 (of an original sample of 1,000) members of Division 29 (Psychotherapy) of the American Psychological Association (Pope et al. 1979). Respondents were asked: (1) if they had engaged in sexual intimacies, as students, with their psychology educators; (2) if they had engaged in sexual intimacies, as educators, with their students; and (3) if they had engaged in sexual intimacies, as therapists, with their patients.

There were significant gender differences in all three areas. An average of 9.4 percent (16.5 percent of the women, 3 percent of the men) reported engaging in sex as students with their educators. About one-half of these instances were with teachers; slightly less than one-half involved clinical supervisors; the few remaining involved administrators. An average of 13 percent (8 percent of the women, 19 percent of the men) reported engaging in sex as educators with their students (including clinical supervisees). An average of 7 percent (3 percent of the women, 12 percent of the men) reported engaging in sex, as therapists, with their patients.

There also appeared to be a significant increase in the educator-student sexual activity over time. One of every four women who had received her doctorate in psychology within the past 6 years reported engaging in sex with at least one of her educators (contrasted to 5 percent of the women who had had her doctorate for more than 21 years). Seventy-five percent of these women indicated that they had engaged in sex with a teacher; 47 percent with a clinical supervisor.

Only 2 percent of all respondents affirmed the statement, "I believe that sexual relationships between students and their psychology teachers, administrators, or clinical supervisors can be beneficial to both parties."

Pope et al. (1979), taking account of the varying ratios of women and men in the roles of educator, therapist, student, and client, conclude:

> When sexual contact occurs in the context of psychology training or psychotherapy, the predominant pattern is quite clear and simple: An older, higher status man becomes sexually active with a younger, subordinate woman. In each of the higher status professional roles (teacher, supervisor, administrator, therapist), a much higher percentage of men than women engage in sex with those students or clients for whom they have assumed professional responsibility. In the lower status role of student, a far greater proportion of women than men are sexually active with their teachers, administrators, and clinical supervisors . . . [a pattern] . . . found in previous research on sexual relations between therapist and client. (p. 687)

Robinson and Reid (1985), using a questionnaire similar to that developed by Pope et al. (1979), obtained anonymous responses from 287 women (out of an original sample of 954) chosen randomly from the 1978 membership directory of the American Psychological Association. They focused exclusively on women because of the prior data showing the greater likelihood that psychology educators would engage in sex with female, rather than male, students. It is important to note that they did not select their sample on the basis of divisional membership, and thus their findings are applicable to psychologists generally rather than solely to clinicians.

Sexual contact with an educator was reported by 13.6 percent of the respondents. Of those who reported contact, 76 percent reported sexual intimacies with at least one teacher, 38 percent with at least one clinical supervisor, and 20 percent with at least one administrator. At the time of the contact, most (76 percent) women were less than 24 years of age. Clinical students experienced the highest incidence of sexual contact. There were no significant differences based on marital status.

Almost one-half of their respondents (48.1 percent) reported some form of (attempted) seduction by at least one educator during their years as students. The most common aspect of these attempted seductions was "flirting," reported by 73 percent. Of those female students who experienced seductive behavior by an educator, 86 percent reported an attempted seduction by at least one teacher, 49.6 percent by at least one clinical supervisor, and 27.3 percent by at least one administrator.

Clinical students experienced more attempted seductions than did other students. Younger women were more likely than older women to be the recipients of seductive behaviors. Of those female students who experienced seductive behaviors, 60 percent were married at the time, and 28 percent had children.

Robinson and Reid's study included a second phase focusing on employees (rather than students). The following data represent the opinions of both students and employees. An overwhelming majority (95.7 percent) of the students and employees believed that sexual relationships with their educators and employers were likely to be detrimental to one or both parties. Most (90.1 percent) believed that there should be clearly formulated policies and special grievance procedures (92.4 percent) for incidents involving sexual harassment for students and employees in psychology.

Examining the patterns of response, Robinson and Reid conclude that the data "suggest that the more vulnerable a woman, the more likely she will experience harassment. . . . Vulnerability was found to increase the likelihood that an individual would experience sexual harassment" (p. 517).

Glaser and Thorpe (1986) obtained anonymous responses from 464 (from an original sample of 1,000) female members of Division 12 (Clinical) of the American Psychological Association. In discussing their choice of questions and their limiting the sample to women, the authors note:

> It should be noted that the sex of the educators was not specified anywhere on the questionnaire. Although the great majority of in-

stances of intimacy most likely involves male educators and female students, the authors considered that the ethical problems involved in such contact derive from the power differential in those relationships, not from the gender of the participants. (p. 45)

Their finding that 17 percent reported engaging in intimate sexual contact with one or more psychology educators during graduate training is in close agreement with the 16.5 percent figure reported by Pope et al. (1979).

In 69 percent of the cases, the intimacy occurred with only one educator. Glaser and Thorpe asked the respondent to identify both the primary role of the educator involved in the initial sexual contact and to specify the number of educators in that role with whom the student worked during training. One-third (33 percent) of these initial sexual contacts were with research/academic advisers, while 3.2 was the average number of advisers with whom students worked. A little over one-fourth (27 percent) of the initial sexual contacts were with clinical supervisors, the students reporting an average of 8.9 supervisors with whom they worked. One-fourth (25 percent) of the sexual intimacies were with course instructors, while 16.3 was the average number of instructors. The remaining instances (15 percent) were with "other psychology educators."

Divorce and separation were significantly associated with the likelihood of educator-student sexual involvement. About one-third (34 percent) of those who were divorced or separated—compared to 13 percent who were not divorced or separated—during their training reported sexual contact with at least one educator.

The authors stress that in most cases (62 percent), the intimacy occurred either prior to or during the student's working relationship with the educator.

A large majority believe that sexual intimacy between student and educator is unethical whether it occurs during (96.2 percent) or outside (72.8 percent) the working relationship. Only 2.5 percent believed that such intimacies are not at all coercive if they occur in the working relationship; only 17 percent believed that sex is not at all coercive if it occurs outside the relationship. Most respondents (95.2 percent) believed that sexual contact would have a harmful effect on a working relationship between a student and educator.

Similar to the phenomenon of therapy clients desiring or at least not strongly objecting to sexual contact with their therapists at the time it occurs and only later beginning to realize the coercion and ethical problems inherent in that contact, the respondents in this study who had engaged in sexual intimacies with their educators reported greater awareness now (at the time of the study) of the coercion and ethical problems with the intimacies than at the time they occurred. Most (88 percent) reported that their training programs provided no coverage whatsoever to the subject of sexual intimacies between educators and their students.

Almost one-third (31 percent) of all respondents reported that during their psychology training, they had experienced sexual advances that did not lead to sex. A large minority (42 percent) indicated that they had experienced such advances from more than one educator. While 80 percent had viewed such advances as ethically inappropriate at the time they occurred, 95 percent now viewed those advances as ethically inappropriate. Many reported that the harm from such attempted but unsuccessful seductions was not limited to damage to the working relationship but also included punitive measures taken by the educator against the student. Placing these data in context, Glaser and Thorpe note:

> Neither the nature of those punitive responses nor the sequelae to coerced sex was specified in the questionnaire. However, a few respondents volunteered that they had seriously considered leaving graduate studies in the face of these pressures. By definition, all of the respondents in the present study successfully completed doctoral studies. The profession needs to acknowledge and address the reality of a population of women of unknown numbers who, after gaining keenly competitive admission to doctoral studies in psychology, take leave of that effort and goal not through lack of ability or diligence but through disgust, dissuasion, and misuse. The numbers need not be large for that to be an appalling and shameful situation. (p. 50)

Pope et al. (1987) obtained anonymous responses from 456 (out of an original sample of 1,000) members of Division 29 (Psychotherapy) of the American Psychological Association. The study did not focus on educator-student sexual relationships but asked respondents to indicate their beliefs about 83 behaviors. Relevant to this chapter, 85 percent of the respondents considered sexual intimacies with clinical supervisees to be always unethical, no matter what the circumstances.

ISSUES FOR EDUCATORS

Addressing the problem of educator-student intimacy is long overdue. Mental health professionals must stop pretending that the phenomenon, with its sometimes disastrous consequences, does not occur, or that the availability of students for the sexual enjoyment of educators is a natural perk of the profession. Those struggling to create clear, explicit policies must confront a variety of complex issues, a few of which are listed below. (Some of these have been previously discussed by Pope et al. 1980, 1986.)

First, there is the issue of teaching as a profession. Can a professional relationship be sexualized and still retain its integrity and effectiveness?

> Historically, sexual or, for that matter, familial intimacy has been seen as distorting clear professional judgment. The Hippocratic Oath, for example, prohibits sex between physicians and their patients. Beyond the issue of professional judgment, the professional may be viewed not so much as one who has achieved some high level of useful, specialized skill (an apt description of an accomplished athlete or good plumber), but rather as someone who is accorded special status, income, or security in exchange for which he or she agrees to an ethic of placing the client's interest above all else. A teacher who gains satisfaction for sexual wants or needs through students may have considerable difficulty maintaining the students' interests as primary. (Pope et al. 1980, pp. 157–158)

Second, there is the issue of the possible detrimental effects of educator-student sexual intimacies upon the practice (or malpractice) of the students once they become professionals. Put another way, do training programs that tolerate sexual involvement between students and their teachers foster therapist-patient sexual intimacies? The data collected by Pope et al. (1979) suggested that those who, as students, engage in sexual intimacies with their educators are later at significantly higher risk, as therapists, to engage in sexual intimacies with their patients. Whether this represents some sort of modeling effect or another dynamic can only be speculated at this point.

Third, there is the issue of how educator-student sexual intimacy may affect the degree to which matters of sexual attraction to (as distinct from sexual intimacies with) patients can be openly, honestly, effectively, and safely addressed within training programs. The findings of Pope et al. (1986) suggest that a vast majority (87 percent) of therapists experience sexual attraction, and that only 9 percent report that their training or supervision in this regard was adequate (about one-half received no guidance or training whatsoever).

> Students need to feel that discussion of their sexual feelings will not be taken as seductive or provocative or as inviting or legitimizing a sexualized relationship with their educators. . . . Educators must display the same frankness, honesty, and integrity regarding sexual attraction that they expect their students to emulate. Psychologists need to acknowledge that they may feel sexual attraction to their students as well as to their clients. They need to establish with clarity and maintain with consistency unambiguous ethical and professional standards regarding appropriate and inappropriate handling of these feelings. (Pope et al. 1986, p. 157)

Fourth, there is the issue of evaluation. One of the many tasks of professional educators is to assess the strengths and weaknesses of their students, the aptitudes and performance, the progress (or lack of progress) toward the educational goals and objectives. They communicate the results of these evaluations not only directly to the students, as part of the educational process, but also to others in a variety of significant ways: through discussion with colleagues about whether a student should continue in the program, should receive financial assistance, should graduate; through making a permanent record of formal grades; through letters of recommendation to subsequent training programs and prospective employers; and through communications to the state agencies responsible for screening candidates for licensure. Such evaluations, especially when submitted to future employers and to licensing boards, serve an important regulating function created to ensure the safety and welfare of future consumers of the professional's services.

> Sexual intimacy may seriously compromise the disinterest (not lack of interest) crucial to careful, fair, and valid evaluations. The sexual activity may occur in at least two contexts. First, it may be the expression of a profound personal intimacy, as in romantic or passionate love. Second, participation in sexual activity may be traded for academic advancement, as in prostitution or the "casting couch" tradition in the theater. Both the romantic involvement and the business exchange aspects raise serious doubts about what is being evaluated on what basis. Other fields seem to take a much more critical attitude toward the evaluation process. It is, for instance, seen as wrong for the head of

a business to sleep with a member of the regulatory agency that oversees that business, for an athlete to be living with the referee of the events in which the athlete competes, for a litigant to be romantically involved with a judge trying the case, and so on. (Pope et al. 1980, p. 159)

Fifth, there is the issue of the power differential between students and their educators. Competition for admission to, success in, financial aid during, and employment after training programs is in many instances so brutal and the criteria for advancement are so complex and nebulous, that the student is extremely vulnerable. When such factors are operative, can students genuinely feel free to exercise choice about sexual involvements offered by their educators? Knowing that to rebuff an invitation to a sexual relationship may bring about a variety of punishing consequences, what risks does a student take by saying "no"?

Sixth, the fact that female students are at significantly higher risk for sexual contact with their educators (just as female patients are at more risk than male patients for sexual involvement with a therapist) may, in programs which do not have adequate policies and procedures prohibiting the practice, invite individual and class action suits alleging sexual discrimination (a concept separate from sexual harassment).

ISSUES FOR STUDENTS

The mental health professions obviously need to put their house in order where educator-student sexual intimacies are concerned. But until there are clearly articulated and enforced policies that protect the individuals participating in the training and the integrity of the training process itself, what steps might be usefully considered by students who feel bribed, coerced, and exploited, or who are otherwise uncomfortable about actual or potential sexual involvement with their educators?

First, try to make your decisions on the basis of truly informed choice rather than reflex or a sense of inevitability. Read all you can in this area. Try to analyze the various contingencies. Once you've educated yourself and considered what seem to be all the possible alternatives, you may still feel that, given the practical realities of your program, you are in an intolerable dilemma, faced with what has often been termed a choice between "integrity and survival." But informing yourself as completely as possible is a necessary first step.

Second, keep a log. Document your experiences. If you feel a clinical supervisor is making suggestive comments to you, write down the conversation as close to verbatim as possible as soon as you can after the supervision session.

Third, try to overcome any sense of isolation you may be experiencing. Those who experience rape-response syndrome, therapist-patient sex syndrome, reactions to child abuse, and reactions to spouse battering frequently report having persistent feelings of isolation. They may feel as if they are the only person in the world facing that situation (even if intellectually they know this not to be so), they may feel an irrational sense of shame or guilt that they are in this situation, and they may fear the criticism of others. Try to share your concerns with at least one trusted friend. If possible, make yourself part of a trusted network of people who are truly sensitive to these issues. Unfortunately, you may feel it necessary to find this friend or network outside your training program.

Fourth, it is important in all cases to respect your own feelings. If you are uncomfortable with what you experience as seductive behaviors from one of your educators, that is an important reaction and should be dealt with adequately. Don't ignore or discount that reaction. However, while respecting your feelings, you can also ask yourself if there is a reasonable chance that you misunderstood what the professor said or misinterpreted the behavior?

Fifth, if after gathering as much information as you can and thinking through the situation as carefully as possible, you are convinced that the educator acted unethically with you, do you believe that other students might also be at risk with that educator? Your answer to this question may be of importance in determining under what circumstances you will be confident that the problem has been adequately resolved.

Sixth, does the situation safely permit you to attempt resolving the difficulty privately and directly with the educator?

Seventh, if you do not think it wise to attempt resolving the difficulty directly and privately with the educator, is there some other way you would feel safe trying to address the problem adequately through dialogue with the educator? For example, is there another faculty member whom you would trust to mediate a session between you and the educator during which you would attempt to address the problem?

Eighth, find out about the departmental or university grievance procedures. It is important to obtain solid information—generally from those who have had firsthand experience trying to use these procedures—not just about how they are supposed to work (or how they work "on paper"), but about how they really work.

Ninth, explore other avenues for resolving such dilemmas. In some cases, professional ethics committees may be useful.

Tenth, if you have any question about what your legal rights and recourses are in regard to this dilemma, consult a qualified attorney who is knowledgeable in this area.

CONCLUSION

In failing to address adequately the phenomenon of educator-student sexual intimacies, we do a disservice to our students, to our tasks as educators, and to the integrity of our profession. In some sense, we may be at the point with educator-student sex that we were with therapist-patient sex 20 years ago when the scope of the problem was not generally acknowledged, when the professional ethics codes lacked an explicit prohibition of therapist-patient sex, when therapist-patient sex syndrome and the other harmful sequelae had not been systematically identified, and, perhaps most significantly, when the civil suits resulting in multimillion dollar judgments for plaintiffs (along with much publicity for the defendants and large increases in malpractice premiums for practitioners more generally) had yet to explode upon public consciousness and professional conscience.

Chapter 14

Sexual Boundary Violations of Clergy

William E. Hulme, Ph.D.

The Rev. Jack Morrison was the epitome of the successful pastor. He was the senior pastor of a prestigious church, both in the community and in his denomination. He was well liked in the congregation and respected in the community. People in the community who did not belong to his congregation referred to it as "Rev. Morrison's church."

Jack had married well. Ellen was attractive and talented and worked as hard as Jack with the congregation. But their couple devotions had slipped. Both were too tired and exhausted in the evening when they normally had their devotions. Their sexual relating had also slipped for the same reason. There were occasions when Jack had anticipated sex with Ellen, but by the time they retired to bed the desire seemed to be lost in fatigue.

Jack really did not know where Ellen was. They had not talked about their sexual diminishment or even about their devotional apathy. Jack occasionally asked himself why he did not talk about these things with Ellen. Was it shyness? Or was it fear? Yet they had not been talking about much of anything of late. They passed each other but hardly stopped. They even joked about this with their parishioners and friends. "I'll tell Jack if and when I see him," Ellen would say. Jack lightly remarked that Ellen had said she needed an appointment to see him. They were rutted in a routine.

Another problem for Jack was that he was nearing 45. For some reason 45 had an ominous ring to it. Perhaps because he was approaching 50.

When Mrs. Quinn asked for an appointment after church, Jack took it matter-of-factly. It often happened that someone wanted to speak to him after his sermon. When Mrs. Quinn arrived, she said that Jack's sermon on developing our potential in Christ had left her depressed. "I'm not developing—period," she said. Her marriage had been a mistake, she said. Her husband had been very persuasive, and she had been very young. But they had little in common. He was a sports addict and inveterate bowler, while she liked music and the arts.

Nor had they ever had a good sex life. As she described her lack of a satisfying orgasm and her husband's frequent premature ejaculation, Jack became aware that he was finding her attractive. He had listened to similar descriptions before, but the way in which Mrs. Quinn moved her hands, pursed her lips, and inflected her voice was a unique experience for him.

Although Jack was puzzled by his reaction, he found it pleasant; and needing some pleasure in his life at this time, he continued to see her. She, of course, was deeply grateful for his time and interest. She told him so as they stood together preparing to part. "I just want to hug you," she said—and did. Jack was thoroughly elated. From then on he anticipated this affectionate closure.

Jack knew the relationship was changing from pastoral counseling to something special. So did Mrs. Quinn. But neither verbalized it to the other. The joy this relationship was giving him moved Jack to dismiss the misgivings that he also had over the relationship. He even found it difficult to acknowledge that the hugs were becoming embraces.

Mrs. Quinn informed him at the close of one of their sessions that her husband was going to his sales convention, her children were at summer camp, and she was going to spend the week at their cottage on a nearby lake. Would he like to see their cottage, and would it be possible to combine the visit with their session next week? Jack's heart began to pound. Impulsively he said, "Why not!"

Jack told his secretary that he would be making calls that afternoon and would not be back in the office. True. When Mrs. Quinn opened the door and received him by extending both hands, Jack felt the excitement of a teenager on his first date. They made a pretense of counseling after touring the cottage. If only she were awakened sexually just once—then she might believe that her dismal sexual life was not all her fault. How good it would be for her to feel like a real woman!

Jack's rationalizing mind was receptive to such altruism. Normally he would have received such a suggestion with amusement: how could anyone but the most naive take it with any seriousness? But Jack was no longer normal. And Mrs. Quinn was right. Jack did awaken something in her she had long doubted existed. He had "ministered" to her in a way only he and she could understand.

According to Jack's rationalized logic, that should have been it. But then they both felt strongly the need to repeat the experience— and to repeat it again. Their new relationship was getting more and more difficult to conceal, but they were pulling it off quite well. Yet Jack knew now that he was hooked. Mrs. Quinn, whom he now called Betsy, and he had justified their activities by their feelings. If what they were doing made both of them feel so good and alive, could it be anything but constructive? Surely God understood.

God did, it seemed, until Jack looked at his wife. Then all of his rationalization crumbled. He knew Ellen would be crushed if she knew. How could he continue with Betsy Quinn? How could he stop? Jack, for the first time, faced up to his pastoral responsibility for his counselee.

Where was divine guidance in this experience that seemed so right because it felt so good? Was it not primarily a problem of chronology? If only he had met Betsy before he met Ellen. Ellen was more his partner in the ministry. Betsy was more his total person mate. But past, present, and future are all one with God. So why should our time problems be so important? This kind of metaphysical reasoning appealed to Jack, but it did little to relieve the stress created by his violation.

WHO IS JACK MORRISON?

As a pastor who has violated a sexual boundary with a parishioner, Jack is typical in two respects. He is male and married. Most clergy are male and married. Also, he is a pastor of a mainline denomination that is neither Catholic nor Eastern Orthodox. This does not mean that Catholic and Eastern Orthodox clergy do not commit sexual boundary violations. It simply means that I am focusing on clergy that I know best.

The ministry in which Jack violated sexual boundaries is pastoral counseling. There are, of course, other ministerial activities in which these violations occur, specifically the co-laboring activities in which clergy minister with other staff members of a congregation, professional or lay. In fact, these co-laboring ministries are probably the scene for more violations than pastoral counseling. I have chosen pastoral counseling because it is the ministry that most closely approximates the functions of the other helping professionals dealt with in this book.

Jack's violation of the sexual boundaries of his counseling illustrates how this violation is similar to those of other helping professionals. The signs of the approaching violation appeared early. Jack's counseling sessions with Mrs. Quinn were under his control. Yet he allowed them to continue long past his usual hour. Also, he took no action to terminate the sessions even though he normally did so because of his concern for creating dependency. Jack was also aware of the stimulation he was receiving from this particular relationship. In fact, his anticipation of these appointments excited him for days beforehand.

There was the usual role of rationalization in pushing back the boundaries as preparation for the violation. His motive, he told himself, was to help the counselee to become free of the weight of her low self-esteem. He resisted whatever sensible warnings he experienced to remove himself from this high-risk relationship. Actually, it was the riskiness of the venture that provided the excitement and stimulation that he had been missing. Always he felt protected by his good feelings. Were they not sufficient justification for what was happening? Jack chose to describe the relationship in these nonresponsible terms rather than taking responsibility for what he was doing.

Then there was the familiar fear of aging that afflicts people as they enter midlife. The terminus of life looms large as death becomes a predator close to home. Two of Jack's seminary classmates had died recently, and he discovered himself reading the obituaries in the newspaper to note the ages of the deceased. While Mrs. Quinn had been married about as long as the Morrisons, she was probably 10 years younger than Jack. His fascinating relationship with this younger woman had diverted Jack's attention from his own aging and death.

Sexual boundary violations can happen to any helping professional, even to the maritally satisfied. But it is not as likely. Jack would not have called his marriage unsatisfactory. The image of clergy protected him. He needed to have a good marriage, and he obviously had one. But the inadequacies of his marital relationship fed into this emotional titillation over Mrs. Quinn. Her entire demeanor "turned him on," activating his subliminal awareness of the deterioration of his and Ellen's relationship. Until now Jack had successfully suppressed this awareness by his workaholic devotion to his ministry.

This was a new experience for Jack. In fact, when it had happened to a neighboring pastor, Jack had little sympathy for the man. But this may not be the case for others of the clergy who violate sexual boundaries. The ministry has its share of sexually disturbed persons who are, in effect, sexual addicts. They love their wives but seem constitutionally incapable of fidelity. They struggle unsuccessfully with themselves to control this addiction. Given the opportunity, however, they seem to have little difficulty in succumbing to temptation.

This addiction afflicts people in all walks of life. Specific political leaders have been notorious in this regard. So also have business executives, psychiatrists, and other therapists. Their positions of authority and power seem to attract those of the opposite sex to provide them their opportunities. There are clergy who have had "close calls" in their boundary violations when their careers could have been ended. But they have been rescued by a forgiving spouse—and sometimes even by a forgiving congregation and bishop. But with all of their promises never again to violate, they frequently slip back into their old patterns because they have an addiction. They need help—from sophisticated counselors and support groups—to achieve their own form of "sobriety."

The clergy as sexual boundary violators are also unique. Their position as clergy goes with a community in which they are the VIPs. It is also a religious community in which the clergy are the symbol bearers of the tradition of faith, specifically, of God. In the decline of the influence of organized religion, I have heard it said that the psychiatrist has become the high priest of our culture. Not so. The psychiatrist, though dealing with problems of the soul, has no community who has ordained him or her to that position and to which he or she is responsible—no community in which he or she is the VIP invested with the symbols of transcendence.

The authority and power implicit in the role of the clergy may elicit sexual responses from some members of the community. The same is true with others in positions of authority whose power and prestige attract. But there is more attraction on the part of some to the clergy precisely because this power and authority has the added dimension of transcendence. The uniqueness of the clergy has several aspects to it.

Sexual Imbalance in the Community

The sexual boundary violations of the clergy are accompanied, if not supported, by a sexual imbalance in the community. The church is predominately peopled by women while the clergy are predominately men. This latter imbalance may soon change as increasing numbers of women are entering the profession that was once closed to them. But as of this writing, there continues to be a preponderance of males among clergy.

There is no such indication, however, that the sexual imbalance in the worshipping community will change. Religion in our culture seems to appeal more to women than to men. This is probably due to the conflict between the independence mystique of the macho image and the dependency posture inherent in religion. To be openly religious a man must take issue with the manly facade of self-sufficiency, which is still difficult to do in our society, although there have been changes here also. While the women's movement may not be drawing women to church, a corresponding men's liberation may well do so.

As things currently exist in the church, male clergy have their preponderant contact with women, whether in staff relationships, in organizational projects, or with counselees. The pastor's counselees are more likely to be women for the same reason that there are more women than men in the faith community. It takes an admission of dependency—or needing help—to seek counseling.

In being a symbol bearer who meets the dependency needs, particularly of women, the male clergy may see themselves as protectors of these dependent people, as a source of strength for them, which may appeal to the male vanity in ways that are not always healthy. The source of strength is someone special, particularly when that source connects with the divine. Ordinary rules may not always apply to those who are special.

Exacerbation of the Offense

The unique context and role of the clergy as the symbol bearers of the faith exacerbates the offense of sexual boundary violations. The offense is obviously present also in secular psychotherapy violations, but because of the community context of the pastor's office, the offense is more extended. The members of the faith community count on the clergy to be "safe," as they do also with psychotherapists and physicians. When they share their needs with the clergy, work together on projects with them, and even share their appreciation in warmly affectionate ways, they have a reason to believe in secure boundaries.

In contrast, clergy who violate these boundaries may interpret their sexual arousal for a woman parishioner as an indicator that the women is desiring them sexually. This may well be a male delusion. The woman more likely may be expressing her sexuality in a safe place. At least this is where it would end if the clergy did not interpret it otherwise.

To betray the trust that the community places in its symbol bearer has serious consequences not only for the persons involved, but also for the entire community. The security and even identity of this community is shaken by clergy violations of sexual boundaries that were deemed safe and secure. People may find their own faith shaken when the symbol bearer of this faith whom they trust betrays that trust. So the offense is aggravated because of the unique and spiritual context of the community within which the clergy function.

Legalistic Upbringing

There is a good possibility that clergy have come from religious homes and backgrounds where legalistic distortions of Christianity made sex largely a matter of law and guilt. Unfortunately, this expression of sex has too often characterized the religious atmosphere of our country. This approach to sex influences people to develop an ambivalent attitude toward their own sexual nature. Behind the legalistic "Don't you dare!" is the secret desire to dare: "I want to." Emphasizing the negative aspects of sex may create within a person a secret desire to be "naughty."

Another reaction to the legalistic suppression of sexual desire is finding an outlet for the hidden ambivalence in fantasy. But because of a law-oriented approach to sex, these fantasies, while giving free rein to the ambivalence, tend to increase one's sense of guilt over sex. But it is a secret guilt, since no one knows about the fantasies. The exception is God, which does not help in integrating one's religious life with one's sexual desires.

One can deal cognitively with sex in a healthy way but emotionally can still be locked into ambivalences formed in one's developing years. We are shaped emotionally by our relationships more than by our formal education. Evidently Jack had an ambivalence over sexual behavior that had been successfully contained, perhaps even unconsciously so, until Mrs. Quinn provided the needed stimulus at the right time in Jack's life to activate it into consciousness.

Since Jack had matured into adulthood, the sexual liberation movement had penetrated all of our society, including the church. When people became liberated from their legalistic backgrounds, their conception of God also was liberated. For those with a legalistic approach to sex, God is a critical parent in this area. Liberation from this critical parent often swings to the opposite extreme. God is then the indulgent parent. What is missed in this liberation is God as a nurturing parent whose love can also be tough. For "liberated" legalists, all rational and even biblical objections to pushing back the boundaries can be pushed aside by the new experience of freedom to say, "I want to."

Wanting to is enough reason to do. When one's image of God is that of an indulgent parent, the problems that would be raised by God as a nurturing parent are rationalized away. What emerges in this liberated state is the spoiled child syndrome in which one seeks to manipulate the structures to get what one wants. The fact that Jack was very persuasive as a minister and could move people to do as he wished probably influenced him to think he could do as he wished in his relationship with Mrs. Quinn. When one is gifted in persuasive abilities, it is a real temptation to exploit this gift for one's own self-aggrandizement.

Special Protection

Given a special place in the community, the symbol bearer may assume a special protection. Rules are necessary but perhaps not for the symbol bearer. Subliminally, self-indulged clergy may believe that they will be spared the consequences of violating boundaries. The familiar example is the pastor's driving. Laypeople like to joke about it. "The way our pastor drives, you have to believe God is looking out for him," they say. So if God—the indulgent parent—is looking out for him, he can afford to take chances—he can violate the limits. The person who is special stands out rather than fits in.

This same mindset may extend also to sexual limits. Clergy are special in God's community. As the VIP of the congregation with a place next to God, clergy have exceptional status. Those who see themselves as special may not like denying (taking a "no" to) their desires. God—the sentimentalized indulgent parent—will make an exception for special me. This is the "mama-daddy's boy" logic. Not wanting to deny one's desires also goes with the liberation movements in our culture, particularly the sexual liberation movement. When this liberation mindset is adopted by a specially indulged divine symbol bearer, we have the potential for the scandals that have marred television evangelism. But the wayward television evangelist is only the extreme of this predisposition for boundary violations to which clergy in general are susceptible.

The symbol bearer's peril is self-inflation. He or she has the authority associated with divinity to speak and to do. For those lacking in inner security, the door is open to a spiritualized megalomania. Moral standards are OK, but my—our—case is an exception. Is this the way Jack rationalized his behavior? "My intentions in breaking the rules were good." "I was attempting to help Mrs. Quinn discover her God-given potential." His was a justification by good intentions, which is a far cry from justification by grace.

Even in such self-indulged rationalizing, however, boundary-violating clergy feel the need to be subtle about their behavior. In spite of their state of self-inflation, there is still a need for self-deception. The facts are too crass at their face value: "You are screwing one of your counselees in violation of a moral code you have promised not only to uphold but also to exemplify." This would be too much. So the need is for a graduating process. First, actions are rationalized in terms of feelings, and then God is rationalized in terms of feelings. What feels good and makes the other feel good is sentimentalized as God-blessed. In all of this subtle buildup of justification, there is little if any reference to the objective biblical base of the faith community. The Bible is more easily avoided than rationalized.

One's liberated refashioning of God's image may convince one that God understands. There is safety in this assurance since we are in control of our image of God. But God is beyond our control. We cannot even control the image of God held by the people of a congregation. They may not be as understanding. If these violations were known, the symbol bearer might not be as persuasive as heretofore. That specter had entered Jack's mind. He could see the faces of his trusting council as he sought to explain his actions, but they were not smiling.

The process of boundary violations began long before Jack actually transgressed these boundaries. It began when he failed to hold to his own limits in the length and frequency of the counseling sessions. By failing to observe these limits, Jack showed that he had already made the choice for a different kind of relationship. He had decided to take the risky road. The actual boundary violation was an occasion waiting to happen. Jack consistently resisted facing what he could have seen, namely, the purpose behind his decision to make a difference in his counseling relationship with Mrs. Quinn.

People in high-stress vocations feel the need for a distraction from the stress. A sexual dalliance on the side, as it were, may provide this distraction. The parish ministry can be a high-stress vocation. Several, including myself, have written on this subject to suggest ways to manage stress in the ministry. Consequently, one cannot overlook the possibility that job stress can be a contributor to sexual boundary violations of clergy.

A sexual dalliance works better than most distractors. Taking a vacation or a holiday may remove one geographically but not psychologically from the source of stress. But the excitement of a sexual encounter combined with the risk of the boundary violation is too much even for stress. But as a distraction the sexual encounter is also a deception. One returns from vacations and holidays, but as Jack discovered, one does not "return" from a sexual boundary violation. It simply does not end as vacations do. Both parties in the violation are likely to get hooked and to want more and more.

There is also a loneliness in the clergy profession. The office of the ministry goes with a community in which the clergy have high status. How then can they be lonely? Being a symbol bearer in the community can also set one apart from the community. Only the clergy share this distinction. The other side of being a VIP is the loneliness that goes with the status. The clergy spouse can also be lonely in the congregation. Many assuage this loneliness by having jobs outside the congregation where they meet others with whom they do not have an exceptional status.

Some clergy seek to assuage their loneliness by throwing themselves into their work. Many clergy, however, develop friendships with other clergy in the locality. But if one senses envy among one's peers, as Jack did, it is difficult to form friendships with them. Some clergy also develop genuine friendships within the congregation in spite of their pastoral responsibilities for these people.

Being a VIP in the congregation means that clergy are easily adulated. People need an ideal, somebody better than they are; and when this ideal includes the values of religion, they strongly desire their pastor to be such a model. People are often quite aware of their own weakness of faith and need to think of the pastor as one whose faith is strong.

By the same token, clergy are easily criticized. When their clay feet are obviously revealed, the congregation's disappointment may show itself in attack. Authority figures who carry the high expectations of the people need to "walk circumspectly," lest they offend their followers. St. Paul put this responsibility onto all Christians. "But fornication and all impurity or covetness must not even be named among you, as is fitting among the saints" (Ephesians 5:3). But Christians have tended to put this responsibility primarily on their clergy.

The clergy, like other authority figures, inherit the authority problems of some of their people. Since clergy are symbol bearers for God, they can become the scapegoat for God for those who are angry about their lot in life, but who find it difficult to blame God directly. Also some people have an antipathy for authorities, and the clergy may be their convenient target. Laypersons have been known to joke about having "roast preacher" for Sunday dinner.

Both adulation and criticism are hard to take for the symbol bearer. It is difficult not to begin to believe the adulating praise if one constantly receives it. The self-inflation that follows may set one up for unrealistic expectations. On the other hand, when the criticism becomes excessive, one's self-esteem can deteriorate. The discouragement that follows may set one up for unrealistic distractions.

Clergy work with volunteers. Most of them are a pleasure to work with. Some of them, however, are unreliable. It would be convenient to be able to discharge them, but this is usually not an option. Others are self-appointed critics. If clergy have difficulties with these volunteers who are a problem, they develop strained and frustrating relationships with the very people they must depend upon to maintain the parish program. Jack had his share of these difficult people. They are one of the major sources of clergy stress.

Clergy tend to be pleasers. They want to fulfill the expectations of their people. For Jack, pleasing paid off. People responded to his pleasing ways by rewarding him with respect and affection. But for others, it may not work. The more they try to please, it seems, the more they get dumped on. This should not happen according to the "contract" under which people-pleasers function. For their pleasing and even self-sacrificing ways, they are supposed to be rewarded with praise and support.

Many people-pleasing authorities are passive-aggressive by nature. Their accommodating approach hides their aggressiveness. But when the "contract" is violated, their aggressiveness may come to the fore. They become angry, feel sorry for themselves, and lay guilt trips on the transgressors.

But even if the people-pleasing system works, it can lead to spouse displeasing. Making sacrifices and accommodations in time and energy for people in the congregation can leave the spouse with the short end of this time and energy. Clergy who find it difficult to say no to their people create a triangular situation for their marriage that is potentially destructive. Many spouses are reluctant to complain because their clergy spouses are in such demand by the congregation. So they begin to resist the congregation. Most of them make their own adjustments to being on the short end of the spouse's stick, but do so at the expense of both their own and their spouse's emotional satisfaction.

So being sexually titillated by someone other than one's spouse can appeal to the emotionally isolated pastor as a quick fix for aggravating frustration. The ambivalence over one's sexual desire may be just under the surface. The triangle—already there in principle—is now personified in a sexually attractive person of the parish. But now the destructive nature of the triangle is no longer contained.

The sexual violation becomes a source of excitement and pleasure that provides a balance to an overdose of work that has become a pain. No doubt some pastors need a balance. We can hardly prosper when our emotional needs are denied. But choosing this way to balance one's life with pleasure only seduces one into further imbalance. For the chosen pleasure itself soon becomes pain.

PREVENTIVE EDUCATION AND CARE

To prevent these tragic violations of sexual boundaries by clergy, the church needs to begin at the beginning, namely, in theological education. This preventive education includes classroom discussion of the possibilities of these violations for each student. As a seminary professor of pastoral care, I have had my share of former students who have violated these boundaries. I have made it a point to talk with them when possible, sometimes even through a counseling relationship. What I learned from them I pass on to my present students.

But seminaries need to go beyond the classroom to fulfill their responsibility for the prevention of these boundary violations. One of my colleagues, together with his spouse, conducts marriage care groups for our married students. I, with my spouse, conduct spiritual growth workshops. Too often seminary students believe that their relationship problems will pass once they finish seminary. They do not. It is in seminary, if not before, that students need to confront problems in their relationships with themselves, their spouses, their fellow students, and with God. The seminary community, which includes administrators, faculty, and students, needs to draw from its own resources the kind of help that is needed for a total-person education for the ministry.

This same kind of total-person support needs to be a part of the continuing education of clergy as this is provided by seminaries or by denominational administrators of clergy conferences. The ministry as well as other professions need this continual support in order to deal constructively with all the exigencies of this fascinating but at times frustrating vocation. This support and nurture is needed also for clergy spouses who are profoundly affected by these violations of sexual boundaries.

While sexual distortions are primarily emotional and formed in early years, they can be diminished and repaired by reeducation programs that deal also with feelings. This reeducation begins with the basic principle that sexual attraction is normal and God-given, even sexual attraction to those other than one's spouse. The moral values involved in freedom of decision lie beyond the attraction, which is simply a spontaneous response to a pleasing stimulation.

Our cultural approach to sexuality would agree that sexual attraction is normal, but would also say that when sex is available and desired, the natural response is to take it. It rarely takes into consideration the legitimacy of a moral decision. Human responsibility seems not to go beyond the instinctual reactions of the lower animals. This interpretation of sexual attraction and desire is obviously not much help in preventing violations of sexual boundaries. Even the word *violate* implies responsibility.

Charles Rassieur in his book, *The Problem Clergymen Don't Talk About* (1976), quotes a pastor in regard to a woman counselee, "Hey, she turns me on! I wonder what's going to happen now?" (p. 71). Anybody who has to wonder about this is ill prepared for any vocation in which responsibility is expected. This is a question that needs to be faced and resolved when one accepts the call to be ordained. It is a question of identity. If you know who you are, you will not wonder what will happen when you become turned on by another with whom you are involved in a ministerial function. You will know.

Since this particular pastor does not know what will happen now that a counselee has turned him on, he is showing that he is not prepared for reality or for the acceptance of those limits that go with his confession of faith. He seems hooked by a parent-child tension over his sexuality that has prevented his maturation into adulthood. All such turn-ons call for decision, commitment, and identity. If these have not been sufficiently formed in regard to one's sexuality prior to the occasion, one has good reason to wonder what will happen.

But when you have faced your options and have dealt honestly with ambivalences, including sexual desires as well as personal goals, and have made the necessary decisions and commitment that identify you as an adult with your own value system, then you can be at ease with yourself rather than living in fear of your unidentified and therefore unpredictable ambivalences. You can trust yourself to keep to the limits that you have faced and accepted. You know who you are and therefore have little reason to play games with yourself in which you subtly identify with an alien part of yourself in order to bypass the acceptable part.

Such "adult" clergy can deal openly with the phenomenon of transference in their counseling and, therefore, can prevent it from generating into a countertransference to which they succumb. Christian clergy serve a Lord who was moved with compassion to reach out and to heal. Compassion is one of the noblest of human attributes, but it can also lead to passion, even as sharing our pains leads to a bonding with the one who listens.

As an example of such bonding, a woman counselee with a troubled marriage may say to her pastoral counselor, "I wish I could talk to my husband like I can talk to you." The pastor obviously feels flattered by this tribute to his counseling. But if he knows who he is, his response will be congruent with his identity. "This is our goal—for you to talk with your husband as you talk with me—and this is what we are working toward." This response does not put the counselee down for her compliment, nor does it fix her in her transference; rather, it structures for her the nature of the counseling relationship and its purpose and informs her clearly where the pastor is. The pastor has remained on firm ground for the counselee. Needing his strength at the moment, she knows now that she is safe with him.

But if the pastor should respond within himself to the counselee's flattering remark: "And I wish I could talk to my wife like I can talk with you," a countertransference reaction is also taking place. The pastor is in a precarious position for himself, his counselee, his spouse, his counselee's spouse, and his congregation. His ambivalence about his role with the counselee is coming to the surface. He is already failing her as a counselor.

Faced with a possible violation of a sexual boundary, this pastor needs to act. His relationship to the counselee will no longer be therapeutic, professional, or priestly if he continues to meet his own needs for intimate communication through her. Unless he takes action to control his countertransference, the relationship is potentially destructive.

The first of his needed acts is to begin to bring his own involvement as a counselor with this woman to an end. It is time for referral. Of course she will object. But he is the counselor. He can explain truthfully that he has done what he can for her and it is time now to get more expertise. He can offer to arrange the referral for her.

His next action is to get help for himself and for his marriage. Perhaps the two can be done together, depending on his spouse's cooperation. It is time for an honest sharing with his spouse about the need for them to work together in their marriage with a counselor so that they might regain the intimacy and communication they both need for an emotionally satisfying relationship.

The pastor also needs help for his spiritual condition. He needs to share his dissatisfied state of mind with a pastoral counselor who can assist him in refocusing on his identity and calling both as a person and as a pastor.

CONCLUSION

There is a risk in taking on the responsibility of any helping profession. The office of the ministry is no exception. There are many occasions for frustration and discouragement as well as for elation and satisfaction. There are also occasions for acting out in destructive ways whatever ambivalent desires we have. The depressing potential of frustration as well as the inflating potential of elation make us susceptible to destructive activities. Clergy are in general unsupervised. They plan their own hours in their work and plot their own activities. They work behind closed as well as open doors. The protection that clergy and the congregations have in this unsupervised ministry is the commitment of the clergy to their calling, the accepting attitude of the clergy toward their own sexual passions, and the wholesome respect of the clergy's responsibility for their own actions.

Chapter 15

Sexual Contact in Fiduciary Relationships

Shirley Feldman-Summers, Ph.D.

The term *fiduciary relationship* is not widely used outside the legal profession. Nevertheless, most people who offer medical, mental health, and legal services can readily understand what is implied by that term—that is, it refers to a special relationship in which one person accepts the trust and confidence of another to act in the latter's best interest.

As defined by Black's Law Dictionary (Black 1979), a fiduciary relationship exists: "where there is special confidence reposed in one who in equity and good conscience is bound to act in good faith and with due regard to interests of one reposing the confidence" (pp. 753–754).

There is no doubt that physicians, psychiatrists, mental health counselors, and attorneys are "fiduciaries." People in these professions as a matter of course hold themselves out as worthy of the trust and confidence of their patients or clients, and routinely profess that they are bound to act in the best interest of those who seek their services.

It may be argued that other professionals, such as teachers, should be included under the heading of "fiduciaries." That is, it may be argued that students—even college students—often place trust and confidence in their teachers in a manner similar to that observed in, say, a therapist-client relationship, especially when the teacher is sought out for individual guidance and assistance.

It is well known that there has been growing concern about the frequency with which fiduciaries—such as psychiatrists or psychologists—either promote or allow the relationship with a client to be transformed into a romantic or sexual one. Numerous articles have been published in professional journals on the subject, some focused primarily on the ethics or legality of the practice, and others focused on the impacts of the practice on the client and/or the therapeutic relationship. Similar interest has recently been shown in sexual relationships between graduate students and their professors (Robinson and Reid 1985). Interest in the subject appears to be somewhat less in other professions, though it could not be said that sexual contact does not occur in these other professions. For example, attorneys who have engaged in sexual relations with their divorce clients have been subjected to disciplinary sanctions.[1] Moreover, as this chapter will demonstrate, sexual contact in the context of these other forms of professional relationships is similar in its dynamics and impact to that between therapist and client.

The aims of this chapter are threefold: to explore the reasons why sexual contact occurs in fiduciary relationships, to examine the psychological impacts of sexual activities in fiduciary relationships, and to discuss the ethical and/or legal implications of such activities between a fiduciary—such as an attorney or a psychotherapist—and a client.[2]

When appropriate, empirical findings and/or theoretical analyses published by others will be supplemented with observations based on the author's clinical experience with women who have had sexual contact with one of the following: a mental health counselor, attorney, gynecologist, chiropractor, psychiatrist, or high school teacher.[3]

THE REASONS

A fiduciary relationship ordinarily involves a social interaction between two people. It is elementary that when trying to discover the causes of a particular kind of behavior in a social interaction— whether sexual or otherwise—one must examine the characteristics of the people involved and the characteristics of the situation. Hence, as a point of departure we look to the client, the fiduciary, and the circumstances.

The Client

The available data, including case studies, suggest that clients who have been involved in sexual contact with a fiduciary tend to have two features in common: first, they are likely to be women, and second, they are likely to be psychologically vulnerable.

As for gender of the client, the surveys of mental health professionals cited in Chapters 1–3 suggest that far more women than men report having had sexual contact with their psychotherapist. The survey cited in Chapter 13 that investigated sexual contacts between graduate students in psychology and their professors or supervisors also revealed a significant gender difference.

Reports of males who have been sexually involved with their psychiatrists or their teachers are rare, as are reports of male sexual involvement with their attorneys or their physicians. Although sexual involvement can obviously occur in cases involving a male client, the prevalence of such involvement is apparently low.

As for vulnerability, it may be argued that there are two major factors to be considered, namely, the presence of a preexisting condition, and the operation of the transference process. As shown below, both sources of vulnerability diminish the likelihood that a client will be able to resist his or her own urges or the advances of the fiduciary.

Preexisting condition. In principle, any kind of psychopathology that interferes with judgment, or that diminishes the client's ability (or desire) to make rational decisions, can and probably does, render the client vulnerable. In practice, however, there appear to be two major sources of psychological vulnerability insofar as sexual contact with a fiduciary is concerned: an overriding need for approval or acceptance and a state of psychological dependency. Either the need for approval or the state of dependency may be transient (i.e., due to a specific set of circumstances). They also may be sufficiently long-standing or generalized as to be regarded as characterological.

It is generally assumed that a strong need for acceptance or approval is linked to low self-esteem or low self-worth (Dittes 1959). Low self-esteem, in turn, can be attributed to a history of rejection (actual or perceived) by persons whose positive regard is sought or valued (Rogers 1959).

Common sense tells us that a person who has suffered many years of physical abuse by a spouse, for example, is likely to have very low self-esteem, and empirical studies support that view (Hilberman and Munson 1977–78). By the same token, a person who has recently experienced rejection by a loved one (e.g., through divorce) may experience—at least on a short-term basis—very strong feelings of low self-worth (Santrock 1983). Moreover, there is reason to believe that a traumatic event—such as rape or childhood molestation—can produce strong and enduring feelings of self-doubt or lack of self-worth (DeFrancis 1969; Myers et al. 1984).

Common sense also suggests that individuals who suffer low self-esteem will probably have positive feelings toward someone who treats them as though they are "worthy" or "valuable." For example, a client with chronically low self-esteem can be expected to develop an attraction toward a therapist who offers assurances that the client is a "good person."

Our common-sense predictions are supported by numerous studies conducted from the standpoint of reinforcement theory, which states in its simplest form that we tend to be attracted toward people who reward us (Berscheid and Walster 1978; Byrne and Clore 1970; Lott and Lott 1961). Furthermore, there is evidence to suggest the following relationship between self-esteem and attraction: the lower a person's self-confidence or self-esteem, the greater the attraction toward someone who shows interest or acceptance (Dittes 1959; Jacobs et al. 1971; Walster 1965).

Cases in which clients have developed a strong attraction toward their health care provider often involve women with low self-esteem that can be attributed to a history of abuse. The cases of M.G. and O.M. are illustrative.

> M.G. is a 49-year-old elementary schoolteacher, who sought treatment after having had sexual intercourse with her gynecologist. She had a history of sexual molestation and emotional abuse by her father. Her mother was cold and distant and rarely intervened on behalf of her children when her husband became angry and abusive. M.G. reports having had few friends as a child and adolescent, and feeling like a "throwaway." Shortly after completing high school, she married the only man who had expressed an interest in her. Her husband eventually began to denigrate her by referring to her as "stupid" and "ugly" and calling her "a clumsy farm girl," and he would periodically abuse her physically, particularly during his alcoholic binges. After 30 years of marriage, she felt unloved, unwanted, and mistreated. She was open to the flattery and professions of caring made by her gynecologist, who made his first sexual advance during the course of a gynecological exam.

A quite different history resulted in a similar state of psychological vulnerability in the case of O.M.:

O.M. was a 27-year-old married mother of three when she first met the psychiatrist with whom she eventually developed a long-term romantic relationship. She was the 5th of 10 children in a poor rural family. Her father was an alcoholic who became threatening and unpredictable when he drank. Her mother bore the brunt of her father's abuse and held the view that women were to be compliant. O.M. rebelled against that view and was seen as being different from the rest of the family. She was molested by her brother-in-law when she was about 10 years old and was later molested by one of her high school teachers. She never told anyone about either experience until she was in therapy. When she was 18 years old, she met and fell in love with a married man. Throughout their relationship, he told her that he didn't love his wife and planned to divorce her. Although she believed him, she felt betrayed by him when he urged her to have sex with his brother. Shortly after she refused, he was killed in an automobile accident, after which her feelings of guilt, confusion, and abandonment were intensified. O.M. was the only one of her siblings to go to college, but she was forced to quit college after 1 year when she developed rheumatoid arthritis. During this year, she met the man she later married, became pregnant by him, but aborted the fetus.

After marriage, O.M.'s life became even more difficult: Her husband showed little affection, was chronically unemployed, and on several occasions left her and their children without warning, sometimes for weeks at a time. By the time her third child was born, O.M. was feeling depressed and overwhelmed. She saw herself and her life as worthless. She felt guilty and ashamed about her role in the childhood molestations, the abortion, and her relationships with men. She sought psychiatric help, but her first psychiatrist was a disappointment because he was not sympathetic, but instead told her that she should consider herself lucky, and should "snap out of" her depression. She attempted suicide and was hospitalized. While hospitalized, she came into contact with a different psychiatrist who, in her words, "didn't blame" her for her problems, but instead was sympathetic and emphasized "the good things" about her. He made her "feel good" about herself. When he made a romantic advance in an early session, she felt "accepted."

Both M.G. and O.M. were deeply affected by their long histories of abuse and/or rejection and by other events in their lives that caused them to question their self-worth. They desperately wanted to feel valued and accepted. They particularly wanted to be seen as valuable and desirable by an adult male. When the health care providers by whom they were treated expressed a desire for them in a manner that conveyed love and/or acceptance, it was not surprising that they reciprocated by developing strong feelings of attraction and a willingness to do whatever was necessary to assure a continuance of the interest that had been shown in them. From the standpoint of reinforcement theory, the health care providers in question were "rewarding" in that they satisfied very strong needs felt by their clients.

There is no reason to think that vulnerability due to a need for approval and acceptance occurs only in connection with women who seek health care, as in the foregoing examples. On the contrary, it seems obvious that a person who seeks the services of any type of fiduciary could be suffering from strong needs for approval and acceptance. For example, even a self-assured, well-integrated woman whose spouse has recently left her for, say, a younger woman can be expected to develop strong doubts about her desirability as a mate, her attractiveness, or her self-worth in general, at least on a short-term basis. If her divorce attorney assures her, directly or indirectly, that she is attractive and desirable, we would expect her to develop positive feelings toward him. Simply put, the attorney who provides psychological rewards for his or her vulnerable client will probably be seen in a more favorable light than would otherwise be the case.

A second major source of psychological vulnerability is an exaggerated dependence on the fiduciary in question. That is, the client may feel that the help or guidance of another is crucial, and that without that help or guidance the problem at hand—whatever it may be—cannot be solved.

Dependency can, of course, be situation specific in that it involves reliance only in connection with a particular problem. Dependency may also be a characteristic way of behaving on the part of the client, due to a long history of being encouraged to be dependent. Moreover, it is often suggested that females in particular are encouraged in our culture to be dependent upon (and compliant with) males, especially males in positions of authority (Herman 1981). Some have suggested that women who have dependent personality disorders are simply "overconforming" to sex role stereotypes, (i.e., passivity and a tendency to be subordinate) (Chesler 1972b; Kaplan 1983).

Whether the dependency is situation specific or an underlying characteristic of the client, it appears to have a similar effect in terms of vulnerability. That is, clients find it difficult to resist the advances of the fiduciary because of a fear of losing the assistance of someone on whom they depend (Bouhoutsos et al. 1983). A case example showing dependency-vulnerability is provided by the case of E.R., who was sexually abused by her attorney.

E.R. was 28 years old and married to a physically and emotionally abusive husband. When she sought the help of an attorney, one leg was in a full-length cast due to an injury caused by her husband. The attorney she contacted seemed confident that he could intervene to help her, and she felt that she had found someone who was "powerful enough" to fight her husband. At their first meeting, she gave him a retainer of $500, which was all she had in savings. He told her to return to his office that evening to sign the papers that he was planning to take to the court to obtain a restraining order. When she returned, she found that they were alone in his office. He soon began to make physical contact with her by rubbing her shoulders. He insisted that she let him "massage" her to relieve her tension. She complied, and after persuading her to lie on the floor, moved from her shoulders and back to her breasts. She was shocked, yet felt trapped by the circumstances: He had her retainer; she desperately wanted protection from her husband; and she felt that to resist would leave her unprotected, with no way to retain a different attorney. As she remained frozen with indecision, he partially disrobed her. He then fondled her genitals and performed oral sex on her. He also instructed her to touch his penis and to kiss his nipples. Still feeling "trapped," she complied, and was only able to extricate herself from the situation when she told the attorney that she had to leave because her son was expecting her. She never returned to his office.

Another example of dependency-vulnerability is provided by the case of R.J., who had been taught to be dependent upon males, and to use compliance to avoid conflict. She was 19 years old when her chiropractor had intercourse with her during a treatment session.

R.J. grew up in a traditional household in which her father worked and her mother gave up her own career aspirations to be a homemaker. She was encouraged to develop traditional sex role attitudes. During her adolescence, she was discouraged from becoming independent, especially by her mother. R.J.'s first experience with sexual intercourse occurred in high school when her boyfriend physically overcame her resistance. Even though she felt that she had been forced, and even though sex was almost always painful, she continued to date her boyfriend and to have sex with him for another year and a half.

The episode with her chiropractor occurred when she went to him for treatment for back and neck strain. She knew and trusted him because he had been the family chiropractor for several years. During the second treatment session, he instructed her to wear a gown, and after manipulating her spine and neck, began to massage her legs and calves. He then asked her to turn on her back, following which he began to massage her abdomen, and eventually her breasts and genital area. He then removed her underpants and had intercourse with her. R.J. states that she didn't want to have any sexual contact with the chiropractor, but that she felt powerless to do anything about it once it began. She felt that simply going along with him would avoid the conflict and criticism that she had seen throughout her life when people resisted those in authority. She states, "I didn't know how to resist."

The vulnerability of either low self-esteem or high dependency is compounded if the underlying feelings are revealed to the fiduciary. Having acquired such information, the fiduciary is now in a position to misuse or exploit these "weaknesses" on the part of the trusting client. Enhanced vulnerability due to revelation is virtually inevitable in the therapist-client situation because the client is encouraged to "tell all." Revelation may also be present in cases of other kinds of professional relationships, though the astute nonpsychotherapeutic professional probably needs little self-disclosure. That is, the needs in question are often readily apparent to almost anyone.

As indicated earlier, both low self-esteem and high dependency needs may be short-term and situationally induced. They may also be of long-standing duration and so pervasive as to interfere with every-day functioning, thereby reflecting a personality disorder. In such cases, low self-esteem and high dependency needs would probably be accompanied by other symptoms (e.g., the symptom constellations recognized as borderline, histrionic, or dependent personality disorders) (American Psychiatric Association, DSM-III-R, 1987).

Individuals who have personality disorders tend not only to have strong needs for dependency and approval, but also to have other characteristics that make them especially vulnerable to sexual exploitation by a trusted authority. For example, it is generally recognized that persons with borderline personality disorder have "a pattern of unstable and intense interpersonal relationships characterized by alternating between extremes of overidealization and devaluation," and engage in "frantic efforts to avoid real or imagined abandonment" (DSM-III-R, p. 347). A person with a histrionic personality disorder "constantly seeks or demands reassurance, approval, or praise." Further, "in relationships they attempt to control the opposite sex or to enter into a dependent relationship" (pp. 348–349).

As for a dependent personality disorder, the DSM-III-R states:

People with this disorder are unable to make everyday decisions without an excessive amount of advice and reassurance from others, and will even allow others to make most of their important decisions. . . . This excessive dependence on others leads to difficulty in initiating projects or doing things on one's own. People with this disorder tend to feel uncomfortable or helpless when alone, and will go to great lengths to avoid being alone. . . . These people are easily hurt by criticism and disapproval, and tend to subordinate themselves to others, agreeing with people even when they believe them to be wrong, for fear of being rejected. They will volunteer to do things that are unpleasant or demeaning in order to get others to like them. (p. 353)

The presence of personality disorders in cases of sexual contacts with fiduciaries has not been documented. However, Stone (as cited in Pope and Bouhoutsos 1986) found that women whose prior relationships were characterized by "anxious attachments" were more likely to become sexually involved with their therapists than were women who did not display that characteristic. To the extent that "anxious attachments" reflect a personality disorder—such as dependent personality—Stone's findings support the notion that personality disorders involving dependency and/or low self-esteem contribute to vulnerability.

Transference. The role of transference in therapist-client sexual contact has been extensively discussed in previous chapters and is generally seen as an important contributor to client vulnerability (Pope and Bouhoutsos 1986).

Notwithstanding the diversity of views concerning the importance of transference for therapy, there is little doubt that most clients can be expected to develop strong feelings of love or adoration toward the therapist, obviously rendering them vulnerable to advances by the therapist. The presence of such feelings in cases of therapist-client sexual contact can easily be seen in the following case example from the author's own practice.

V.J. was born and raised on a farm. She described herself as being shy and always afraid. She didn't think her mother loved her and often fantasized about running away to live with her grandmother, whom she saw as more affectionate than her parents. Although she believed her father loved her, she felt ambivalent about him because he often teased and made fun of her. She described her mother as depressed and withdrawn and her father as hard-working but often absent from the home. V.J. did well academically but felt socially isolated. She was married at age 18 and was divorced at about age 25. After two other unsatisfying romantic relationships, she found herself at age 31 becoming fearful "of everything." She began drinking alcohol excessively and experienced blackouts about once a month. She also began having what she called "weird thoughts" and felt more insecure than she had ever felt in her life. She became reclusive and invented excuses to avoid interacting socially. She then sought the assistance of a mental health counselor. She described her first session with him by saying, "I crawled into his office, and I walked out of his office on cloud 9." She eventually saw her counselor as an ideal father, stating "I wished that I had been raised by someone like him." By the time he made sexual advances, her feelings of adoration were at their strongest: "I thought he was like God."

Similar feelings of adoration were reported by O.M., whose case was referred to earlier: When asked to describe how she felt toward her psychiatrist prior to the romantic contact, O.M. said, "He treated me like a human being. He didn't see the negative side of me. I felt close to him like I had never felt close to any man before. He was a god-like creature—someone I idealized."

Although transference is most often discussed in the context of psychotherapy, theorists such as Becker (1973) and Brenner (1982) reason that it can occur with any suitable target. If so, there is no reason why transference cannot occur in the context of an attorney-client relationship, a physician-patient relationship, or a teacher-student relationship. All that is required is an authority figure who bears at least a symbolic resemblance to the actual or idealized other about whom the client/patient/student has unconscious fantasies or unresolved conflicts.

An example of transference in a teacher-student relationship is afforded by the case of C.R., who was a senior in high school when one of her teachers befriended her and eventually drew her into a sexual relationship with him. She was 17 years old.

C.R. reports a generally happy childhood with attentive and affectionate parents. When she entered puberty, however, it seemed to her that her father became increasingly uncomfortable with her sexual maturation, and withdrew from her. She felt rejected and blamed herself. Her teacher, who was approximately the same age as her father, showed her the attention and affection she felt she had lost. She describes him as the kind of father she wished that she had known earlier in her life. To her, he was everything her father was not: charismatic, easygoing, and interested in her. When he kissed her for the first time, she says that she felt like "a little girl," and as though she "had been molested." As they continued to interact, and as he continued to put pressure on her for additional sexual contact, her predominant feelings were of powerlessness: "I felt like I was 6 years old . . . when he started pressuring me for greater sexual contact, I felt helpless to resist. I remember when I was practically completely undressed in his car, I felt like I couldn't move . . . like my wrists had been tied. . . . "

Her words graphically reveal how transference in a fiduciary relationship confers a psychological similarity between incest and sexual abuse.

The Fiduciary

Even with the strongest feelings on the part of the client, sexual contact is unlikely to occur in the absence of a willing fiduciary. Unfortunately, very little is known about the factors that contribute to the fiduciary's decision to engage in sexual activities with a client.

In the therapeutic context, the most common theoretical explanation revolves around the concept of "countertransference" (i.e., a reaction by the therapist to the client's transference). Fundamental to the explanations based on this definition of countertransference is the proposition that the professional in question is suffering from his own psychological problems (e.g., unresolved conflicts) which lead (unconsciously) to positive feelings toward the client. From the analytic standpoint, he acts on those feelings in an effort to obtain the kind of outcome which had not occurred in connection with a "significant person" in his own past.

Although nonanalytic explanations of the fiduciary's behavior are apparently rare (Pope et al. 1986), alternative explanations are certainly available. For example, it may be argued that just as the fiduciary can be "rewarding" to the client, so too can the client be "rewarding" to the fiduciary. That is, by showing respect, adoration, or love, a client may satisfy narcissistic needs of the fiduciary, thereby "rewarding" him or her, and leading to feelings of attraction for the client. These feelings could be sufficiently strong that the fiduciary is unable to resist the urge to act on them.

It may also be suggested that the fiduciary's conduct is influenced at least in part by a belief that if the client is a consenting adult, sexual activity between them is acceptable, notwithstanding the trust relationship that exists. Although sexual activity with clients is regarded as unethical by the professional associations of certain types of fiduciaries (e.g., mental health practitioners), there is no reason to believe that such ethical prohibitions are universally endorsed, even in professions that have long prohibited sexual contact with clients (e.g., psychiatrists and psychologists). It is just as likely that a significant number of all health professionals, for example, believe that adults who are capable of giving meaningful consent should be free to engage in sexual activities, regardless of the relationship between them.[4] In the area of psychotherapy, for example, there have been advocates of sexual contact with clients (McCartney 1966), and it is probably the case that many health care professionals who engage in sexual activity with their clients justify their conduct, at least to themselves, as being helpful or "therapeutic" for the client (Pope and Bouhoutsos 1986).

Finally, in the case of male fiduciaries, predatory sexism may play a role. It has been claimed that our society supports the pursuit of women for sexual purposes and the use of pressure to accomplish that end (Goodchilds and Zellman 1984; Kanin and Parcell 1977; Muehlenhard and Linton 1987). Males who have adopted that view, and who see virtually any woman as legitimate "prey," may find it difficult to resist their urges when faced with a female client, especially when "it would do her so much good."

The Circumstances

The most salient feature of the situation in which sexual contact occurs between a fiduciary and his or her "client" is the fiduciary relationship itself. That is, the situation is characterized by an expectation of trustworthiness, typically encouraged by the fiduciary. Such expectations are also encouraged and supported by societal norms (i.e., we are ordinarily taught at an early age to trust our physicians, for example). Common sense tells us that we are ordinarily slow to resist or even question the suggestions of one who is trusted to be acting in our best interests.

A second salient feature of the situation is the unequal power relationship. The fiduciary—whether a psychiatrist, psychologist, gynecologist, attorney, or teacher—is typically understood to be someone with special expertise and knowledge. People with special expertise or knowledge in our society are ordinarily accorded power and authority by others (Raven and French 1958). We are encouraged to comply with the demands of those in positions of authority, and we learn at an early age that resistance can be expected to produce negative outcomes.

Finally, a third salient feature of the situation is the privacy that typically characterizes the interactions with a fiduciary.[5] Office consultations with health care providers and attorneys ordinarily occur in complete privacy, so there is no one else present to question the contemplated sexual activity or to provide social support to a person who may wish to resist, but "doesn't know how."

Each situation in which sexual contact occurs can and will have its own peculiar features that contribute to the occurrence of the behavior in question. However, the features discussed above are probably sufficient to create conditions that make the sexual contact possible. Simply put, a fiduciary who decides to make advances toward a client (or patient or student) does so under conditions that are particularly conducive to compliance. A client who resists is, at least implicitly, questioning the trustworthiness and authority of the fiduciary and is doing so without any immediate social support. It should not be surprising that a client, especially one who is vulnerable, would be slow to resist.

CONSEQUENCES OF SEXUAL CONTACT

Most reports of the effects of sexual contact in fiduciary relationships concern sexual relationships between clients and mental health professionals, such as psychiatrists and psychologists. These reports generally support the view that sexual contact in the context of a therapist-client relationship is likely to disrupt the therapeutic process and cause harm to the client (Chesler 1972a; Dahlberg 1970; Forer 1969; Hare-Mustin 1974; Holroyd 1983; Masters and Johnson 1970; Siassi and Thomas 1973; Taylor and Wagner 1976; Voth 1972; Whittington 1981).

Several recent studies have documented particular types of negative consequences for the client. For example, Apfel and Simon (1985) "catalogued" the following negative consequences for women who had sexual contact with their therapist, noting that not all the women suffered all of the following problems: ambivalence and mistrust of subsequent therapists, doubt of their own sense of reality, repetition of childhood trauma that became fixated rather than interpreted, bondage to the offending therapist, exacerbated sexual dysfunctions and problems in intimacy with men; guilt and shame associated with the sexual contact; additional difficulties with discussing sexual fantasies in therapy; and feelings of abandonment and disorganization related to the abrupt termination of the therapy.

Very little has been published on sexual contact between clients and fiduciaries other than mental health practitioners. Burgess (1981) described 16 cases involving gynecologists who manually manipulated a patient's genitals "under the guise of conducting an internal gynecological examination" (p. 1336). She reports that all of the women described negative reactions to the gynecological examination, including feeling "dirty, humiliated, degraded, embarrassed, and nauseated" (p. 1338).

In a recent study conducted by this author and Gwendolyn Jones (1984), data were obtained about psychological and psychosomatic symptoms experienced by three groups of women: those who had engaged in sexual contact with their psychotherapists; those who had engaged in sexual contact with a different type of health care practitioner (e.g., plastic surgeon, dentist) while that person's patient; and a third group of women who had been in therapy, but who had never engaged in sexual activities with their therapist or other health care provider. Compared with women who had not had sexual contact with their therapists, women who reported such contact revealed greater mistrust of and anger toward therapists and men in general. They also reported a greater number of psychological and psychosomatic symptoms following termination of therapy. No significant differences were found between the symptoms experienced by women who reported sexual contact with their therapists and those who reported sexual contact with a different kind of health care provider. Finally, the data suggest that severity of impact is significantly related to several factors, namely, the magnitude of psychological and psychosomatic symptoms prior to treatment, prior sexual victimization, and the marital status of the health care practitioner. Specifically, the women who reported the greatest number of posttreatment symptoms were those who had the most severe preexisting problems, or who had been sexually victimized prior to entering therapy, or those whose therapist or other provider was married at the time of their sexual involvement.

Studies designed to identify the psychological impacts of sexual contact between teachers and their students, or between attorneys and their clients, have apparently not been conducted.[6] Even in the absence of empirical data, however, there is reason to predict that such contact carries with it a risk of harm for the client or student, for several reasons.

1. Whenever an attorney or teacher (or any other fiduciary) engages in a romantic or sexual relationship with a student or client, a "dual role" relationship is established. These roles may be entirely incompatible, in that the attorney (for example) may find it difficult to provide objective advice to a client with whom a sexual relationship has been developed. That is, the attorney may be reluctant to provide unpleasant advice out of fear that the client will discontinue the sexual relationship. If so, the client will not receive the quality of service which he or she is entitled to receive, and will be harmed accordingly. By the same token, a teacher who engages in sexual contact with a student may have difficulty evaluating the student's work in an objective manner, in which case the student's education will be adversely affected (Dziech and Weiner 1984; Munich 1978; Pope et al. 1980).

2. A dual role relationship can be expected to create confusion on the part of the client as to the nature of the relationship. If the client is already suffering from psychological problems (e.g., a borderline personality disorder or low self-esteem), the effects of such confusion can be severe.

3. In the event that the client eventually decides that his or her trust has been abused, or that exploitation has occurred, we would expect a decreased willingness to trust others in a similar role. Also, the author's own clinical experience suggests that embarrassment, humiliation, and shame are common reactions to a realization that one's trust has been abused, especially if that realization occurs when it is discovered that the client or student is not "special," but instead is merely one of many who have been (or are) sexually involved with the fiduciary in question.

ETHICAL AND LEGAL IMPLICATIONS

Most national associations of mental health care providers prohibit sexual activity with a client. For example, the published ethical standards of psychologists, psychiatrists, social workers, and pastoral counselors state that sexual activity with a client is unethical.[7] It is generally recognized that sexual activity with a client is a breach of fiduciary duty and renders the practitioner liable for damages in a malpractice suit.[8] The practitioner's employer may also be held liable for damages arising from the sexual involvement.[9]

Not all professional associations expressly prohibit sexual contacts with a client, however. For example, the rules of professional conduct for lawyers as published by the American Bar Association are silent on the subject, as are the ethical standards for chiropractors. Nevertheless, it can be argued that even in the absence of clear prohibitions, a fiduciary should avoid sexual involvement with a client (or student), for the following reasons:

1. It can always be claimed that meaningful consent cannot be given in a situation that is characterized by unequal power. For example, a graduate student who is approached sexually by his or her thesis adviser will almost certainly find it difficult to decline the invitation due to a fear that the professor will withdraw support or will retaliate in some other fashion (Dziech and Weiner 1984). Similar claims can be made in any situation in which unequal power exists. In short, the fiduciary who makes advances toward a client or student is open to a charge of exploiting the other due to the unequal power relationship.

2. Even if consent can be given, exploitation can nevertheless be argued if the fiduciary has acquired information about the client's vulnerabilities that otherwise would remain concealed. For example, a divorce client who reveals loneliness and insecurity to his or her attorney thereby provides the attorney with information that can readily be used to facilitate sexual involvement.

3. It can be argued that a conflict of interest arises whenever sexual involvement occurs in a fiduciary relationship. That is, the client's interest—which should be paramount—may be in conflict with the fiduciary's interest in maintaining the sexual or romantic features of the relationship. At the very least, the sexual involvement will almost certainly detract from the time and energy that otherwise would be devoted to the client's needs. Also, the fiduciary may be disinclined to offer advice that would be beneficial to the client, if that advice would diminish the likelihood of continued sexual contact.

4. Finally, and most important, the sexual involvement creates an unnecessary risk of psychological harm for the client. At the least, the client is likely to experience confusion and doubt as to the nature of the relationship. In the case of clients who have preexisting psychological problems, the risk of severe harm is substantial when they discover that they are not "special," or that the sexual or romantic involvement is not permanent, which is frequently the case (Apfel and Simon 1985; Sonne et al. 1985).

Fiduciaries who are not trained in mental health may not fully appreciate the psychological impacts of sexual contact with their clients. Hence, it may be unrealistic to expect certain types of fiduciaries (e.g., dentists, attorneys) to understand the potential for adverse psychological effects. However, the other three reasons to avoid sexual contact do not require special knowledge to understand; they are accessible to common sense. Fiduciaries who ignore common sense, and ignore the growing concern about sexual abuse of clients, risk harming those who rely on them, and ultimately risk harming themselves and their profession.

Notes

[1] American Bar Association/Bureau of National Affairs. Lawyer's Manual on Professional Conduct. Vol 3. Current Reports, pp. 127–128, 1987.

[2] For the sake of convenience, the trusting individual will typically be referred to as a "client," although in some cases such an individual is a patient or a student.

[3] Pursuant to the guidelines suggested by Simon (1987), all clients whose cases are reported here read and discussed the manuscript before publication and gave written permission to include their materials. Of the eight clients described, only two are now in therapy, and in both instances their cases are a matter of public record because of litigation.

[4] A recent survey of psychologists revealed that 5 percent believed it was ethical to have erotic contact with a client (Pope et al. 1987).

[5] The teacher-student relationship is an exception, at least in high school settings. Professor-student relationships, however, can involve frequent consultations that are private.

[6] Note, however, that Glaser and Thorpe (1986) surveyed female members of the American Psychological Association and found that most of those who had sexual relationships with their professors in graduate school now believe that the experience had "negative effects" on them.

[7] See: American Psychological Association, Ethical Principles for Psychologists, Washington, DC, 1981; American Psychiatric Association, Principles of Medical Ethics, with Annotations Especially Applicable to Psychiatry, 1981; National Association of Social Workers Code of Ethics, 1980; American Association of Pastoral Counselors, Code of Ethics, 1980.

[8] See, for example, *Omer* v. *Edgren,* 38 Wash. App. 376, 685 P2d 635, 1984.

[9] See *Simmons* v. *United States,* 805 F2d 1363 (9th Cir. 1986).

Chapter 16

Medicolegal Aspects of Professional Sexual Exploitation

Irwin N. Perr, M.D., J.D.

The use of the words *sexual exploitation* in dealing with the issues in this book is relatively explicit and clear. Nonetheless, the application of these words to a professional relationship is sometimes fraught with ambiguity—or at the very least, uncertain in application.

Assuming that "sexual" is reasonably well understood, conflict may arise in terms of what constitutes exploitation. Is all sexual contact inherently exploitative? In this era of concern over sexual harassment and male-female relationships, social attitudes become of paramount importance. For example, there are those who believe that all sexual interaction is inherently exploitative—under any circumstance whatsoever.

Human beings are driven by their biological urges, particularly in their younger years. These drives, which may not be inherently evil or socially unacceptable, can become so in the context of certain socially defined relationships. This transformation is especially likely when a defined professional relationship exists—where one party has authority, power, or knowledge and the other party is dependent, trusting, and reliant.

When an abuse takes place, various social instrumentalities may be applied to remedy the apparent defect in acceptable behavior.

These instrumentalities involve the use of the law to punish the wrong-doer (criminal law), to compensate the person who may be perceived as being a victim (civil law), and to remove the authority to practice in the profession (administrative law)—another form of punishment. In addition, each profession may use sanctions to dissociate itself from the wrongdoer. These extralegal professional sanctions may result in a reprimand, probation, or expulsion from the professional group. Such acts by a private group may involve a legal review when the offender fights the organizational action, or reference to the organizational review may be incorporated in one of the three legal procedures mentioned. Hence all involve legal consequences for perceived mis-behavior.

THE EXTENT OF THE PROBLEM

Complaints concerning psychologists' sexual involvement with clients are the leading cause of lawsuits. Sexual involvement by psychiatrists with patients now constitutes the second leading cause of all profes-sional practice litigation. Studies demonstrating the prevalence of such behaviors are reviewed elsewhere in this volume (Chapters 1–3).

A recent book by Burgess and Hartman (1986) has reviewed some of the implications of sexual exploitation, focusing on rather gross examples of abuse and pinpointing many of the problems in-volved both for perpetrators and for patients/clients. Smith and Bisbing (1986) have compiled an extensive review of legal cases involving sexual exploitation by professionals. This notebook-bound collection of cases is a most valuable source for anyone interested in this subject and includes a chapter titled "Sexual Exploitation—Undue Familiarity," which was published in *Medical Malpractice: Psychiatric Care* by Smith (1986). The reader should refer to the Smith and Bisbing work for analysis of specific cases or for use as a resource in reviewing specific cases. However, review of legal cases alone is confusing because the numerous legal theories vary according to jurisdiction and because of the inconsistencies noted from case to case—a problem common in a tort system with 50-plus jurisdictions. Obviously, the large number of cases cannot be reviewed here; the striking fact about most is that they involve very blatant abuses but do not necessarily provide guidelines for all possibilities that might arise.

Smith's report of 1988 brought to 167 the number of cases involving sexual exploitation reported by Smith and Bisbing in their review in 1986. By profession or occupation, these were (1) nonpsychiatric physicians, 59; (2) psychiatrists, 46; (3) psychologists, 17; and (4) other health care professionals (e.g., marriage counselor, physician assistant), 12; (5) chiropractors, 6; (6) dentists, 8; (7) social workers, 3; (8) clergy, 4; and (9) attorney/judge, 12. [These figures are slightly altered to correct errors in addition in the original article.] Sixty-seven of these involved civil suits, 31 were criminal cases, 52 involved professional sanctions, and 18 involved insurance actions only. Claimants were upheld in 117 cases, defendants in 27, and in 24 neither party emerged with a clear victory.

THE ACTORS: PROFESSIONALS

The single group most affected by litigation has been that of nonpsychiatric physicians. Women have been assaulted and raped by physicians, often in combination with the use of drugs. In one case an anesthesiologist was reported to have placed his penis in the mouths of anesthetized patients on more than 160 occasions. Other women have been subjected to impulsive fondling of breasts or genitals in the course of examination or minor surgical treatment. Occasionally the physician has indicated that such fondling was "treatment," but this is uncommon. These assaults generally occur in a medical environment such as an office or hospital room. Chiropractors in particular have had a penchant for unusual forms of massaging and the use of instruments such as vibrating dildos.

A bizarre case was that of *Ross v. State, Div. of Professions* (342 So. 2d 1023, 1977), in which the Florida state board of chiropractors revoked the license of a chiropractor who, treating a back condition, used a vibrator to bring his female patient to orgasm, then straddled the patient and manipulated himself to orgasm. The appeals court reduced the penalty to 6 months because of his 22 years of service in his profession, affidavits about his good moral character, and other supposedly mitigating circumstances. In this case the complaint was of a single incident and was uncorroborated, which raises the issue of sufficiency of proof confronted by courts.

Similarly in a Washington case (*Davidson v. State,* 33 Wash. App. 783, 657 P2d 810, 1983), two patients with low back pain complained of a chiropractor using a vibrator on their breasts and genital areas. He was suspended for 6 months and put on probation for a further 18 months.

Dentists have been involved in a number of assaults. These incidents occurred in an office environment and usually involved bodily contact or penetration, often when anesthesia had been used. Obviously, there is no possible therapeutic implication, and the relationship is not a social one involving competent adults or a relationship that "has gone sour."

No issue of therapy is involved in cases where dentists become involved sexually with patients. Dentists are among the few professional people who utilize anesthesia, and sexual activity utilizing drugs and without consent of the patient clearly violates professional organizational ethical standards, licensing practice codes, criminal statutes, and allowable behavior by civil standards, thereby constituting a tort. For example, in *Melone* v. *State of NY Educ. Dept.* (115, AD 2d 854, 495 NYS 2d 808, 1985), a dentist was charged with professional misconduct for having sexual contacts with five male patients 7 to 15 years of age. His license was revoked.

Psychiatrists have been sued on a significant number of occasions. While there have been incidents involving minors or what might constitute rape, the events have on occasion been that of an evolving "love affair" that ultimately terminates, resulting in litigation by the cast-aside patient. Other psychiatrists have been involved in sexual acts in the course of office therapy and have even charged for their services. Those exploited constitute a varied group, including minors, psychotics, and members of both sexes.

Varying attitudes toward these issues may be found. One major school of thought is directed at what it perceives to be the absolute obligation of psychiatrists not to become involved with patients. In particular, many psychiatrists and some courts incorporate the concept of the misuse of transference as an act of malpractice. This conceptualization may at times be a legal tactic to justify inclusion of sexual exploitation as a misapplication of medical practice (rather than not being considered as malpractice at all), allowing for inclusion of insurance coverage that might otherwise exclude intentional, tortious acts (i.e., acts not accepted as being within professional practice). One may argue that this focus on countertransference is not universally applicable in view of the wide variety of treatment modalities and relationships in psychiatry. For example, if a graduate student has examination anxiety and is seen in two sessions of crisis therapy, does the concept of countertransference necessarily apply to subsequent relationships between the parties?

Psychologists have had legal difficulties similar to psychiatrists and have frequently had their licenses to practice revoked because of sexual activity. Numerous suits for damages have also been filed.

Generally, psychologists have been involved in some type of psychotherapy.

Neither psychiatrists nor psychologists have a monopoly on bizarre personal behaviors. Both have been involved in cases involving couples and marital therapy as well as abuse in situations that involve both training and therapy, especially where the line between education and application is often unclear. Social workers have now joined the group of those vulnerable to lawsuit. In particular, those who practice psychotherapy, counseling, or marital therapy can expect sanctions when abuses occur.

A curious case was that of *Horak* v. *Biris* (474 NE 2d 13, 1985), in which the Illinois appellate court recognized a cause of action of social worker malpractice, overturning a prior Illinois case of 1982, which had refused to allow such litigation. In this case, the social worker had been involved sexually with the wife of a client; he had treated both spouses in marital counseling. In this case, the court stated that the defendant provided "psychological counseling and psychiatric and mental therapeutic care." The court also referred to mishandling of the "transference phenomenon."

Curiously, sex therapists per se do not seem to have been involved in much litigation (see Chapter 11). This is reasonable to the extent that ordinarily psychotherapy and sexual therapy are carefully separated, the purpose of therapy directly involves sexual functioning, and other issues such as impaired competency are not likely to be present.

Considerable potential exists for similar legal involvements for lawyers, judges, clergy, teachers, and others. A small number of cases have involved disciplinary actions against lawyers and judges. The ones against lawyers have involved claims of impropriety in such behaviors as seeking and obtaining sexual favors in return for legal services. In some cases, lawyers have purportedly intimidated wives of criminal defendants to indulge in such activities. One involved a 66-year-old Colorado lawyer who became involved with a defendant's 23-year-old wife, who had "only" a ninth grade education. The wife was described as unduly dependent (*People* v. *Gibbons,* 685 P2d 168, 1984). The court said that sexual misconduct alone would merit censure or suspension, but this and other misbehaviors warranted disbarment. In *State* v. *Heilprin* (59 Wis. 2d 312, 207 NW2d 878, 1973), an attorney blamed touching his clients and exposing himself on a personality disorder and sexual problems in his marriage. His license was suspended until recovery from his mental disorder. Other charges in other cases simply involved what was considered to be unacceptable behaviors, such as touching or exposing oneself. In another case where an attorney stated that his unacceptable behavior was a result of a personality disorder, the court did not accept a "personality disorder" as a defense to a disciplinary proceeding.

In an Indiana case (In re *Wood,* 265 Ind 616, 358 NE2d 128, 1976), an attorney offered to exchange legal services for nude photographs of the client and her daughter. He also had sexual relations with his client. The attorney was suspended from the practice of law for 1 year.

In re *Higgins* (79 AD 2d 145, 436 NYS 2d 71, 1981) an attorney solicited sexual favors from a female in return for favors in his role as judge of the family court. He resigned from the bench, and the Joint Bar Association Grievance Committee upheld a 2-year suspension of his license to practice law.

Similarly, judges have engaged in a variety of analogous behaviors, including vulgarity, grabbing persons of both sexes by various bodily parts, and so forth. Various suits fit in with the now common claim of sexual harassment, and judges have been removed from office for such behaviors.

In Kansas, a judge was censured publicly (removal would have been an appropriate penalty, but he had retired due to a cardiac disability) after having sexual relations with one employee, making demands on another, and terminating employees for refusal to acquiesce to his demands (In re *Hammond,* 224 Kan 745, 585 P2d 1066, 1978).

Smith and Bisbing (1986) noted the case of a Colorado priest who was purportedly sexually intimate with the wife of the plaintiff. The district court dismissed the claim under the First Amendment and indicated that a claim should be made under the Catholic church court system.

THE ACTORS: PATIENTS AND CLIENTS

Sexual involvement between a professional person and a patient or client raises numerous issues, one of which is the competency issue. The competency of the perpetrator is rarely relevant though it has been raised unsuccessfully in defense. To my knowledge, no claims have been made against professionals assumed to be psychotic or incompetent in terms of the usual standards for competency. However, some individuals have claimed that the acts were a result of a personality disorder or situational factors. The courts have generally taken the stance that the mental state of the person is not relevant, which is in conformity with the established law that one cannot defend a tortious act on the basis of incompetency. Such a claim might be applicable to a criminal charge, but I am not aware of the attempted use of such a defense in a criminal court.

The abuse of a relationship with an incompetent patient or client is another matter. Courts have made specific reference to such considerations. Clearly, this would be a factor in assessing damages or even in weighing whether a tortious act occurred (depending on the jurisdiction). Certainly a court or jury is likely to be incensed by actions against a chronically psychotic individual. In one case, a defendant attempted to minimize the damages by claiming that the individual was chronically ill and so was not really harmed. On the other hand, in the *Hartogs* case (*Roy* v. *Hartogs,* 85 Misc. 2d 891, 381 NYS 2d 587, 1976), the court stated that the patient had a long-standing preexisting condition and that she could recover damages only for the aggravation of that condition. Court attitudes seem to have changed considerably since that time.

Clearly any professional person who uses his or her position to sexually abuse a minor, male or female, can find no justification or rationalization for doing so. Depending on the age, criminal sanctions may be applicable, and state licensure boards and professional organizations are not likely to be tolerant in this regard. [I would have to qualify this statement by my knowledge of some situations where state licensure boards imposed rather light penalties, such as short suspensions and probation. It is possible that the boards were concerned about the problems of proof should a full court hearing be held, and so accepted lesser penalties that often are a result of negotiation.]

THE ACTS

The issue of consent in reference to the acts has been discussed above. Consensual acts allow for some degree of disagreement, and the details of the specific situation thus become important. Where there can be no consensual assent by the nonprofessional person, the charge of exploitation becomes more clear.

Where drugs and anesthetics are used, without the assent of the person for the purpose involved, a violation of patient rights could not be more obvious. Similarly, force is not acceptable under any circumstances. In some cases a claim of fraud or sham has been made where women have been assaulted allegedly before they were aware of what was going on.

The acts vary in severity—both by law and in the eyes of decision makers. Sexual remarks, while in bad taste, are not likely to be construed as being particularly harmful or worthy of severe punishment. Kissing and fondling may be quite inappropriate and indeed frightening to individuals who cannot comprehend the motivation or bizarreness in such behavior by a professional person, but the harm is likely to be construed as limited. In a long-term relationship, sexual involvement is compounded by the possibility of dependency and the likelihood that the initial problems are not being reasonably attended to.

Most cases have involved heterosexual acts between professional males and female clients or patients. Claims have involved minors, both male and female. Increasingly, the ranks of professional persons in this country have been augmented by growing numbers of women. It is therefore to be expected that there will be a corresponding increase in the number of females who are charged with exploitation of patients or clients. With homosexual behavior, for example, people have become more accepting of it because of greater exposure to it, but they have also become more willing to openly protest it when they consider it inappropriate.

Two other elements might be considered. One is the tendency current in this country to become more prudish and more sensitive about sexual issues. All forms of sexual activity outside marriage are being questioned, and confusion about relationships abounds. Second, the extreme concern about acquired immune deficiency syndrome (AIDS) has become a factor in the concern over protection for all people exposed to sexual contact under questionable circumstances.

CRIMINAL AND DISCIPLINARY ISSUES

Reference has already been made to the fact that sexual involvement with minors or sexual acts characterized by lack of consent, fraud, or sham may constitute a criminal act everywhere. Because of ambiguity otherwise, some states have taken specific statutory steps to deal with certain forms of professional exploitation.

Several states have criminalized therapist-patient sex. My commentary will not direct itself to acts dealing with minors or adults who may not be able to give consent for reason of mental incapacity. Such rules apply generally throughout the country under the ordinary statutory "rape" or sexual assault standards. In some states, it is required that the offender reasonably know the victim to be a minor or to be of limited mental capacity; in others, lack of knowledge is not a defense. With minors, various age standards may be used. For consent issues, mental retardation is included in the concept of mental illness as referable to this issue (Perr 1968).

In the Minnesota criminal code dealing with sex acts (S.609.341 to 609.351), "psychotherapist" is defined as a physician, psychologist, nurse, chemical dependency counselor, social worker, clergy, or other person, whether or not licensed by the state, who performs or purports to perform psychotherapy. "Psychotherapy" means the professional treatment, assessment, or counseling of a mental or emotional illness, symptom, or condition. "Emotionally dependent" means that the nature of the patient's or former patient's emotional condition and the nature of the treatment provided by the psychotherapist are such that the psychotherapist knows or has reason to know that the patient or former patient is unable to withhold consent to sexual contact or sexual penetration by the psychotherapist. "Therapeutic deception" means a representation by a psychotherapist that sexual contact or sexual penetration by the psychotherapist is consistent with or part of the patient's treatment.

Section 609.344, criminal sexual conduct in the third degree, applies to sexual penetration, and states: (1) the actor (person accused of criminal sexual conduct) is a psychotherapist and the complainant is a patient of the psychotherapist and sexual penetration occurred during the psychotherapy session; consent by the complainant is not a defense; (2) the actor is a psychotherapist and the complainant is a patient or former patient of the psychotherapist and the patient is emotionally dependent upon the psychotherapist; or (3) the actor is a psychotherapist and the complainant is a patient or former patient and the sexual penetration occurred by means of therapeutic deception. Consent by the complainant is not a defense.

Upon conviction, the actor may be subject to imprisonment for not more than 10 years and a fine up to $20,000, or both. Probation may be used if the offender has been accepted by and can respond to a treatment program after professional assessment, in which case the court must also order some incarceration in a jail or workhouse and require that the offender complete a treatment program.

Similarly, criminal sexual conduct in the fourth degree applies to sexual contact, rather than to sexual penetration. Sexual contact refers to intentional touching of the complainant's "intimate parts" and the touching by the complainant of the actor's, complainant's, or another's intimate parts under certain circumstances. Sexual contact also includes touching of the clothing covering the immediate area of the intimate parts. Otherwise the rules regarding psychotherapists under S.609.344 are the same. The penalty is less: a maximum incarceration of 5 years and a maximum fine of $10,000, or both. With a second or subsequent offense within 15 years, a minimum imprisonment of not less than 3 years is mandated.

Minnesota also has a specific statute dealing with a civil cause of action for sexual exploitation (148 A.01-.05). The law defines "emotionally dependent" as noted previously except that it does not refer to sexual penetration; "sexual contact" is sufficient. It defines "former patient" as a person who was given psychotherapy within 2 years prior to sexual contact with the psychotherapist. "Sexual contact," as defined in this statute, as compared with the 609 definitions, includes sexual intercourse, cunnilingus, fellatio, anal intercourse, penetration of genital and anal orifices by the therapist's body or objects, and similar intrusion into the psychotherapist's body by the patient or former patient. It also includes kissing or touching of the body. Sexual contact also includes requests by the therapist for such conduct, and it is applicable whether or not there is consent. It excludes such physical activities upon the patient's body if such acts are part of "standard medical treatment."

A cause of action exists if the sexual act occurred during the period of psychotherapy or afterwards, if the former patient was emotionally dependent on the psychotherapist, or if the sexual contact occurred by means of therapeutic deception. Sexual contact outside a therapy or treatment session is no defense.

Employers may be liable in two situations: (1) if the employer fails to take reasonable action when the employer knows or has reason to know that sexual contact has occurred, and (2) if the employer fails or refuses to make inquiries of employers or former employers about possible sexual contact where such prior employment as a psychotherapist occurred in the last 5 years. The former employer may also be liable if the former employer knew of such contacts, received an inquiry from another employer, or prospective employer, and failed to disclose such contacts. Liability requires that such failure was a proximate and actual cause of any damages (whatever that means). There can be no cause of action against an employer or former employer who complies in good faith. Discovery is limited to the plaintiff's sexual history only if it is relevant and if it is not prejudicial. An action must be commenced within 5 years after the cause of action arises. These rather drastic statutes have apparently not resulted in any particular increase in reported abuses.

One of the interesting questions raised concerning psychiatrists is the limitation to psychotherapy. It is not clear whether the statute applies where other treatments may be utilized to the exclusion of psychotherapy. Therefore, one cannot discern whether diagnostic appraisal or organic therapies in the absence of psychotherapy would subject a physician to inclusion.

Michigan has a statute entitled "Sexual intercourse under pretext of medical treatment" (750.90). This statute applies to any person who undertakes medical treatment of any female person, representing that it is necessary or beneficial to her to have intercourse with a man and shall induce her to have sexual intercourse with any man not her husband. Such a therapist is guilty of a felony and subject to imprisonment up to 10 years. This statute applies only to limited circumstances—to female patients who are involved in heterosexual intercourse—and excludes lesbian or male homosexual acts as well as female therapist–male patient interactions.

In Florida's medical practices act (S 458.331), sexual misconduct in the practice of medicine means violation of the physician-patient relationship through which the physician uses such relationship to induce or attempt to induce the patient to engage or attempt to engage the patient in sexual activity outside the scope of the practice or the scope of generally accepted examination or treatment. Sexual misconduct in the practice of medicine is prohibited.

Under S. 458.331, grounds for disciplinary action, is included exercising influence within a physician-patient relationship for purposes of engaging a patient in sexual activity. A patient shall be presumed to be incapable of giving free, full, and informed consent to sexual activity with his or her physician. In one case, the notation that a psychiatrist's conduct in engaging in a sexual relationship before he had properly terminated the psychiatrist-patient relationship warranted revocation of his license (*Solloway* v. *Department of Professional Regulations,* 421 So. 2d 573, 1982, review denied 430 So. 2d 452).

New Hampshire (Chapter 632-A) includes, as aggravated felonious sexual assault in its criminal code (632-A.2), sexual penetration where the actor engages in the medical treatment or examination of the victim in a manner or for purposes which are not medically recognized as ethical or acceptable.

Wisconsin, in its statute (S. 940.22), defines a "therapist" as a physician, psychologist, social worker, nurse, chemical dependency counselor, member of the clergy, or other person whether or not licensed by the state who performs or purports to perform psychotherapy. Any person who is or holds himself or herself out to be a therapist and who intentionally has a sexual contact with a patient or client during any ongoing therapist-patient or therapist-client relationship, regardless of whether it occurs during any treatment consultation, interview or examination, is guilty of a Class D felony. Consent is not a defense.

INSURANCE AND RELATED LEGAL ISSUES

Professional persons seek to protect themselves from the vagaries of tort litigation by obtaining malpractice insurance. More accurately, such insurance should be called professional liability insurance that covers causes of action in addition to malpractice. Certain peculiarities are inherent in such insurance. For example, protection from claims due to motor vehicle accidents while engaged in professional activities will be covered by automobile insurance. Driving is not a professional act in these circumstances.

Insurers often place limitations on malpractice insurance. Hence, acts that are intentional and harmful and are not ordinarily part of professional practice may be excluded from coverage. Some insurers will state in their policies that they will not cover damages due to sexual activities.

The professional person may find himself or herself in a peculiar position. The insurer may refuse to provide a legal defense with the claim that no malpractice is involved in a sexual exploitation case. However, a claim may be totally unmerited or even fabricated for a variety of motives. A disgruntled patient or ex-patient may utilize the litigation system to express anger or revenge. For example, a paranoid patient may become involved in such litigation, or a hysterical patient may misinterpret the relationship with the therapist. In such cases, the professional person can legitimately claim that the litigation arose from and is a risk of the practice. For this reason, some insurers, such as those for the American Psychiatric Association, will defend a claim, but will not pay for damages if the case is lost.

Sexual misbehavior carries an emotional impact, and juries, in considering damages, may consider sexual abuse to be an extremely willful and wanton misuse of a professional role. As a result, they may impose punitive damages that far exceed the compensatory damages, which may be minimal. Punitive damages are designed to punish misbehavior, and many insurance policies will exclude coverage for such damages.

Many professional persons work for groups, corporations, or governmental entities. The person claiming injury may sue the hiring agency under the doctrine of respondent superior ("let the superiors or higher-ups take care of it"). Agencies and institutions may have a "deeper pocket," and my impression is that juries generally have little sympathy for corporate or governmental entities. On the other hand, sexual abuse is not reasonably to be considered an activity in the ordinary line of duty.

Many government agencies will not be responsible for gross, willful, or malicious behavior not performed in accord with job duties. This policy seems to make sense. Rape is an act of an individual, and the punishment and/or compensation policies should be directed at the individual who commits the act. Certainly taxpayers might question governmental responsibility in such a case. Because of the law in this regard, plaintiffs have attempted to circumvent these rules by claiming that the agency was negligent in hiring the perpetrator and is therefore responsible. Alternatively, they may claim that the agency was negligent in not providing supervision that would have prevented or minimized the injury.

Other philosophical differences may be involved. Some, in defense of those abused, feel that insurance exists to protect the needs of injured parties, not to protect the vulnerability of a professional person to litigation, even though it is the professional who must bear the economic burden. Others state that the tort system really is a punishment system wherein the offender must make amends by financial compensation to those injured. Ironically, the insurance system protects the offender when it insulates the offender from financial punishment. Not only that, the insurance system makes those who committed no wrong financially responsible. Thus one could argue that the insurance system itself may be contributory to wrongful behavior by protecting individuals from the consequences of such behavior.

As readers of case law will discover, damages vary tremendously—from trivial amounts to awards in the millions. No particular logic or reason seems to apply to the assessment of damages even in meritorious cases (this criticism, of course, applies to the entire tort system). As a result, insurance coverage has become increasingly costly, and it is for this reason that some insurers have limited coverage with the assent of the professional associations whose members they insure.

Lastly, courts interpret insurance contracts very rigidly in favor of those covered so that exclusion clauses must be clearly written lest a court order the insurer to provide legal protection or to pay for damages granted.

An early case was that of *Zipkin* v. *Freeman* (436 SW2d 753, 1968), a Missouri case where the doctor made trips with the patient, engaged in nude swimming, arranged group trips with patients, had intercourse with the patient, and was involved in business transactions. The insurance company attempted to avoid defending the doctor or paying any damages on the grounds that the actions were not professional services. The court ruled that the patient was not treated properly and that transference was mishandled, thus being sufficiently related to professional services. One judge carefully indicated that the behaviors did not constitute malpractice: "We note that one does not conduct an illicit adventure with a woman over a period of months through negligence, professional or otherwise."

In *L.L.* v. *Medical Protective Co.* (122 Wis. 2d 455, 362 NW2d 174, 1984), the court similarly upheld coverage for a psychiatrist who had engaged in fellatio with his female patient during therapy sessions. The court adopted the *Zipkin* reasoning concerning treatment that should have been provided.

The *Hartogs* case involved the alleged treatment of a lesbian with "fornicatus Hartogus." One of the suits (*Hartogs* v. *Employers Mutual Liability Ins. Co. of Wisconsin,* 391 NYS2d 962, 1977) involved the question of insurance coverage. The court ruled that fornication therapy did not constitute malpractice because it did not derive from medical practice. The court refused to "indemnify immorality and to pay the expenses of prurience." Coverage for the cost of defense was denied.

The *Hirst* case (*Hirst* v. *St. Paul Fire & Marine Ins. Co.,* 106 Idaho 702, 683 P2d 440, 1984) involved a nonpsychiatric case in which a physician became sexually involved with a high school student. The court ruled that "professional services" did not include all forms of physician conduct, but that the insurance carrier was obligated to provide a defense even if it was not under an obligation to pay damages. A similar result occurred in *Standlee* v. *St. Paul Fire & Marine Ins. Co.* (107 Idaho 899, 693 P2d 1101, 1984).

The *McCabe* case ruling (*Aetna Life* v. *McCabe*, 556 F. Supp 1342 ED Pa., 1983) held an insurance carrier liable for intentional sexual misconduct but not for punitive damages. The policy covered injury from the rendering of or failure to render services with no distinction as to unintentional or intentional acts. The court said that public policy prevented coverage for punitive damages.

The *Smith* case (*Smith* v. *St. Paul Fire & Marine Ins. Co.*, 353 NW2d 130, Minn., 1984) is an example of a case of a physician who was sexually involved with three male minors. The lower court stated that the damages were a result of withholding services and thus professional. The court overturned this decision, ruling that the acts did not represent medical treatment but "were solely for the satisfaction of the doctor's prurient interests."

Insurers were held responsible for damages in a case involving a gynecologist (*St. Paul Fire & Marine Ins. Co.* v. *Ashbury*, 149 Ariz. 565, 720 P2d 540, 1986) and in another involving a psychiatrist (*Vigilant Ins. Co.* v. *Kambly*, 319 NW2d 382, Mich., 1982). The latter seems a bit bizarre because of the specific exclusion in the policy for legal expenses for an alleged criminal act.

In *St. Paul Fire & Marine Ins. Co.* v. *Mitchell*, 296 SE2d 126, Ga., 1982), the appeals court stated that manipulation of the transference phenomenon (as in *Zipkin*) involved a professional service. A similar result occurred in *Vigilant Ins. Co.* v. *Employers Ins. of Wausau* (626 F. Supp, 262, SDNY, 1986).

It should be added that breach of contract and fraud have been other grounds for suit. The penalty for breach of contract is minimal compared to tort verdicts—the cost of services provided or not provided.

ETHICAL ISSUES

All helping professions take a strong stance against involvement by therapists with patients. The ethics committee of the American Psychiatric Association in April 1985 added the following three special annotations to the Principles of Medical Ethics:

Section 1, Annotation 1. The patient may place his/her trust in his/her psychiatrist knowing that the psychiatrist's ethics and professional responsibilities preclude him/her gratifying his/her own needs by ex-

ploiting the patient. This becomes particularly important because of the essentially private, highly personal, and sometimes intensely emotional nature of the relationship established with the psychiatrist. (p. 3)
Section 2, Annotation 1. The requirement that the physician conduct himself/herself with propriety in his/her profession and in all the actions of his/her life is especially important in the case of the psychiatrist because the patient tends to model his/her behavior after that of his/her therapist by identification. Further, the necessary intensity of the therapeutic relationship may tend to activate sexual and other needs and fantasies on the part of both patient and therapist, while weakening the objectivity necessary for control. Sexual activity with a patient is unethical.
Section 2, Annotation 2. The psychiatrist should diligently guard against exploiting information furnished by the patient and should not use the unique position of power afforded him/her by the psychotherapeutic situation to influence the patient in any way not directly relevant to the treatment goals. (p. 4)

The American Psychiatric Association has prepared a statement entitled "Facts About: Patient-Therapist Sexual Contact" for transmission to patients and has provided the mechanism by which complaints may be made.

As this book goes to press, the Assembly of the American Psychiatric Association has endorsed a further modification of the Principles of Medical Ethics. This change specifically addresses the issue of sexual relations with former patients:

Sexual involvement with former patients generally exploits emotions deriving from treatment and therefore almost always is unethical.

The American Medical Association Council on Ethical and Judicial Affairs states: "Sexual misconduct in the practice of medicine violates the trust the patient reposes in the physician and is unethical." This wording apparently allows for deliberation about what constitutes misconduct.

The American Psychological Association Ethical Principles (1981) state:

Principle 6
    a. Sexual intimacies with clients are unethical.
Principle 7
    d. Psychologists do not exploit their professional relationships with clients, supervisees, students, employees, or research partici-

pants, sexually or otherwise. Psychologists do not condone or engage in sexual harassment.

Similarly, the ethical code of the National Association of Social Workers (1980) states in II 5: "The social worker should under no circumstances engage in sexual activities with clients."

CONCLUSION

I have attempted to review in a noncomprehensive fashion many of the legal issues that arise when sexual exploitation of patients or clients by professional persons occurs.

Examples of the various types of litigation have been presented. The professional person who sexually abuses a patient may be subject to numerous sanctions. He or she may be charged with violation of professional ethical standards and faced with reprimand, probation, or suspension. Such behavior may result in loss of other privileges (such as hospital rights, credibility, or status in a courtroom) or inability to obtain other privileges. Organizational action may also be used as an indication of a failure to conform to acceptable professional standards and used as evidence in a civil trial or licensure review.

Exploitation may result in loss of licensure or, at least, in disciplinary action by a licensing board. In addition, those who become involved may be faced with criminal charges under general laws (rape, sexual assault, molestation of a minor) or specific criminal charges in those states that have adopted special legislation referable to therapists.

The intricacies of the tort system have also been summarized with presentation of a few examples. The complexities facing insurers and the economic burden on the professions have become significant elements in American life.

Lastly, the problems of applying ethical rules and determining the boundaries of acceptable behavior have been presented. Review of recent medicolegal cases indicates that the cases that have reached legal review almost uniformly reflect gross abuses of behavior for which there can be no justification. The increasing recognition of the problem also dictates that professional people and professional organizations must develop a keen sensitivity to actual and potential abuses, both in protecting professional autonomy and status and in protecting those who seek help in the atmosphere of trust, reliance, and special knowledge that should characterize professional services.

Afterword

Carol C. Nadelson, M.D.

This book places sexual exploitation in professional relationships within the spectrum of abuse and victimization. It is a serious violation of the boundaries of the professional relationship, and for those experiencing it, a traumatic life event. This problem, as the book emphasizes, pervades a range of professional relationships and fields. It exploits those who enter into these relationships based on expectations of trust. The authors of these chapters have explored the complex dimensions of a problem that cannot remain underground; it violates the basic conceptual tenets of the professions.

Many have questioned the wisdom of being overinclusive and considering teacher-student or teacher-trainee interactions in this category. There are, however, important reasons evolving from the concept of transference to underscore the seriousness of the problem to include the spectrum from harassment to specific sexual involvement, and to emphasize the need for professions to clearly define their boundaries and expectations for ethical behavior.

Perhaps the most controversial issue explored in the book is determining when the therapeutic, teaching, or fiduciary relationship ends and when another kind of relationship is possible. There are major differences of opinion on this subject, ranging from those who feel that it never ends to those who would like to define a specific time frame after termination. However this question is ultimately resolved, it is clear that elements of transference exist in all professional relationships. The nature of these professional relationships implies that providers assume a responsibility to impart expertise, knowledge, advice or wisdom, or to utilize specific skills to help those requesting it. Thus, whether it is a client seeking legal advice, a student enrolled in a course, or a patient requesting medical treatment, the obligation taken on by the provider is to honor this commitment and to assume the responsibility for maintaining the boundaries of the relationship and for honoring the contract implied to the best of his or her ability.

That those who are in dependent positions, such as patients, parishioners, students, and clients, develop transference feelings that affect their interactions in the relationship is evident. The imparting of confidences and fantasies to the minister, the lawyer, or the therapist often affects the ability of patients, parishioners, students, or clients to perceive exploitative aspects of the relationship or to report them. The victim who calls attention to the problem is likely to be blamed and to experience shame and guilt about her participation. If she chooses to stand up to her betrayer publicly, she must face the added burden of being labeled unreliable and emotionally disturbed, especially if she had sought psychiatric treatment. She is also publicly exposed. This loss of privacy can further victimize her. The student whose grade depends on the instructor's judgment or the employee whose evaluation depends on her employer's report is often in a situation where the refusal of a sexual advance risks compromise of her academic or employment status.

This type of abuse and victimization produces repercussions that may not differ substantially from those experienced by victims of other traumatic life events such as rape and incest. They call upon an individual's capacity of mastery in unique and specific ways. Timing of the event, whether it was solitary or repetitive, its relationship to other life stresses, individual personality and situational factors, and the kinds of environmental supports and resources that are available are factors that affect the individual's response. The degree of threat and the perception of control or lack of it are also important variables. There is no accurate way to predict an individual's response immediately or even long afterward.

As with all sexual abuse, the repercussions can be lifelong. For those who are children or adolescents, their picture of the adult world and their own self-concepts change. They are alone, inexperienced, and deceived by someone they trusted. They are helpless to understand and deal with a frightening and confusing experience, and their veracity is often questioned. Adults who are emotionally disturbed or mentally ill also experience similar problems related to deception and helplessness, but since they often come into the relationship with a damaged self-esteem, they are even more vulnerable to this kind of abuse and suffer more serious consequences.

Long-standing symptoms and the development of posttraumatic stress disorder have been reported following other types of sexual abuse. Follow-up studies of abuse victims (Kilpatrick et al. 1979; Nadelson et al. 1982) indicate that, among other symptoms, a substantial percent of women continue to have fear, terror, anxiety, and depressive symptoms, as well as changed sexual attitudes and relationships for a substantial period of time. For many women, posttraumatic symptoms have been reported to increase over time. These women often delay seeking treatment in part because they fear retribution. They also may take longer to define the events that transpired as sexual assault.

The phenomenon described as learned helplessness (see Lystad 1986), the perception of an inability to effect change, has been described as occurring particularly in women. It often keeps them in abusive situations. Those women who continue to see an abusing doctor, lawyer, or clergyman, and even to pay their bills, may be exhibiting this type of behavior. The mistrust and low self-esteem of many of these women also may make it difficult for them to establish trusting relationships with others. In fact, they may have initially sought help because of these problems. They may have sought a confidant and a trusting "parent" in the therapeutic relationship, magnifying the experience of deception and reinforcing the belief that they have no basis for trust. They are often unaware of the rage they harbor because of the long-standing suppression of their fears of loss of control and the assault they experienced on their self-esteem. It is often difficult for these women to report sexual exploitation because they feel that they are on trial. At times, the knowledge that others have had similar experiences is supportive in the disclosure and in seeking help.

This book, the product of authors from different disciplines, explores these issues as they affect individuals in different fields, considers therapeutic approaches, and reaffirms our professional responsibilities and commitment. While clinicians often feel that sexual exploitation in professional relationships is a rare problem and one that does not affect them, the data presented suggest that the problem is serious and certainly more prevalent than most assume. If clinicians are to understand their patients and to be able to elicit accurate histories that may reveal painful and traumatic events many would prefer to keep underground, they must be aware of this problem and its implications, clinically, legally, and ethically.

References

American Bar Association/Bureau of National Affairs Lawyers' Manual on Professional Conduct. Vol 3: Current Reports. Washington, DC, American Bar Association, 1987

Alexander F, French J: Psychoanalytic Therapy. New York, Ronald Press, 1946

American Association of Sex Educators, Counselors, and Therapists: Code of Ethics. Washington, DC, American Association of Sex Educators, Counselors, and Therapists, 1979

American Medical Association, Division of Survey and Data Resources: AMA Physician Masterfile for 1983. Chicago, American Medical Association, 1985

American Psychiatric Association: Principles of Medical Ethics with Annotations Especially Applicable to Psychiatry. Washington, DC, American Psychiatric Association, 1981

American Psychiatric Association: The Principles of Medical Ethics with Annotations Especially Applicable to Psychiatry (1985 ed). Washington, DC, American Psychiatric Association, 1985

American Psychiatric Association: Diagnostic and Statistical Manual of Mental Disorders (Third Edition–R). Washington, DC, American Psychiatric Association, 1987

American Psychological Association: Report of the task force on sex bias and sex role stereotyping in psychotherapeutic practice. Am Psychol 30:1169–1175, 1975

American Psychological Association: Ethical principles of psychologists (rev). Am Psychol 36:633–638, 1981

American Psychological Association: If Sex Enters Into the Psychotherapy Relationship. Washington, DC, American Psychological Association, 1987

APA malpractice claim types constant, but frequency, costs have doubled. Psychiatric News, November 4, 1983, p 3

Apfel RJ, Simon B: Patient-therapist sexual contact, I: psychodynamic perspectives on the causes and results. Psychother Psychosom 43:57–62, 1985

Apfelbaum B: The ego-analytic approach to individual body-work sex therapy: five case examples. Journal of Sex Research 20:44–70, 1984

Arentewicz G, Schmidt G (eds): The Treatment of Sexual Disorders. New York, Basic Books, 1983

Armitage P: Statistical Methods in Medical Research. Oxford, England, Blackwell, 1971

Bajt TR, Pope KS: Therapist-patient sexual intimacy involving children and adolescents. Am Psychol (in press)

Barnhouse RT: Sex between patient and therapist. J Am Acad Psychoanal 6:533–546, 1978

Becker E: The Denial of Death. New York, Free Press, 1973

Bennett BE: Information about your professional liability program (letter). Washington, DC, American Psychological Association Insurance Trust, December 15, 1987

Berscheid E, Walster E: Interpersonal Attraction, 2nd ed. Reading, MA, Addison-Wesley Publishing Co, 1978

Black HC: Black's Law Dictionary, Revised 5th ed. Edited by Nolan, JR, Connolly MJ. St. Paul, MN, West Publishing Co, 1979

Borenzweig H: Touching in clinical social work. Social Casework 64:238–242, 1983

Borys DS, Pope KS: Dual relationships between therapist and client: a national study of attitudes and practices. Professional Psychology (in press)

Borys DS, Meyer CB, Falke RL, et al: Dynamics of treatment groups for victims of therapist sexual misconduct, in Sexual Exploitation of Patients by Health Professionals. Edited by Burgess AW, Hartman CR. New York, Praeger, 1986, pp 178–184

Bouhoutsos JC, Brodsky AM: Mediation in therapist-client sex: a model. Psychotherapy: Theory, Research and Practice 22:189–193, 1985

Bouhoutsos J, Holroyd J, Lerman H, et al: Sexual intimacy between psychotherapists and patients. Professional Psychology: Research and Practice 14:185–196, 1983

Bouhoutsos J, Holroyd J, Lerman H, et al: Mediation in therapist-client sex: a model. Psychotherapy 22:189–193, 1985

Brenner C: The Mind in Conflict. New York, International Universities Press, 1982

Briggs D: The trainee and the borderline client: countertransference pitfalls. Clinical Social Work Journal 6:133–146, 1979

Brodsky AM: Is it ever o.k. for a therapist to have a sexual relationship with a former patient? Paper presented at the mid-winter meeting of Division 12 of the American Psychological Association, San Diego, CA, January 1988

Brown F: Erotic and pseudoerotic elements in the treatment of male patients by female therapists. Clinical Social Work Journal 12(3):244–257, 1985

Buckley P, Karasu TB, Charles E: Psychotherapists view their personal therapy. Psychotherapy: Theory, Research and Practice 18:299–305, 1981

Buie DH: The abandoned therapist. International Journal of Psychoanalytic Psychotherapy 9:227–231, 1982–83

Burgess AW: Physician sexual misconduct and patients' responses. Am J Psychiatry 138:1335–1342, 1981

Burgess AW, Hartman CR: Sexual Exploitation of Patients by Health Professionals. New York, Praeger, 1986

Butler S: Sexual contact between therapists and patients. Unpublished doctoral dissertation, California School of Professional Psychology, Los Angeles, 1975

Butler S, Zelen SL: Sexual intimacies between therapists and patients. Psychotherapy: Theory, Research and Practice 14:139–145, 1977

Byrne D, Clore G: A reinforcement model of evaluative responses. Personality 1:103–128, 1970

Calef V, Weinshel EM: A note on consummation and termination. J Am Psychoanal Assoc 31:643–650, 1983

Carlson R: After analysis: a study of transference dreams following treatment. J Consult Clin Psychol 54:246–252, 1986

Chesler P: Patient and patriarch: women in the psychotherapeutic relationship, in Woman in Sexist Society. Edited by Gornick V, Moran BK. New York, Basic Books, 1971, pp 251–275

Chesler P: The sensuous psychiatrists. New Yorker Magazine, June 19, 1972a, pp 52–61

Chesler P: Women and Madness. New York, Avon Books, 1972b

Claman JM: Mirror hunger in the psychodynamics of sexually abusing therapists. Am J Psychoanal 47(1):35–40, 1987

Collins DT, Mebed AK, Mortimer RL: Patient-therapist sex: consequences for subsequent treatment. McLean Hosp Journal 3(1):24–36, 1978

D'Addario L: Sexual relations between female clients and male therapists. Unpublished doctoral dissertation, California School of Professional Psychology, Los Angeles, 1977

Dahlberg C: Sexual contact between patient and therapist. Contemporary Psychoanal 6:107–124, 1970

Dahlberg C: Sexual contact between patient and therapist. Medical Aspects of Human Sexuality 5:34–56, 1971

Davidson V: Psychiatry's problem with no name: therapist-patient sex. Am J Psychoanal 37:43–50, 1977

DeFrancis V: Protecting the Child Victim of Sex Crimes Committed by Adults. Denver, American Humane Association, 1969

Deutsch H: The Psychology of Women: A Psychoanalytic Interpretation, Vol 1. New York, Grune & Stratton, 1944

Dittes J: Attractiveness of group as function of self-esteem and acceptance by group. Journal of Abnormal and Social Psychology 59:77–82, 1959

Durré L: Comparing romantic and therapeutic relationships, in On Love and Loving: Psychological Perspectives on the Nature and Experience of Romantic Love. Edited by Pope KS. San Francisco, Jossey-Bass, 1980, pp 228–243

Dyer AR: Ethics and Psychiatry. Washington, DC, American Psychiatric Press, 1988

Dziech B, Weiner L: The Lecherous Professor: Sexual Harassment on Campus. Boston, Beacon Press, 1984

Edelson M: The Termination of Intensive Psychotherapy. Springfield, Charles C Thomas, 1963

Edelstein L: The Hippocratic Oath: Text, Translation, and Interpretation. Baltimore, Johns Hopkins University Press, 1943

Ethics Committee of the American Psychological Association: Report of the Ethics Committee. Am Psychol 41:694–697, 1985

Ethics Committee of the American Psychological Association: Trends in ethics cases, common pitfalls, and published resources. Am Psychol 43:564–572, 1988

Federn P: Ego Psychology and the Psychoses. New York, Basic Books, 1952

Feldman-Summers S, Jones G: Psychological impacts of sexual contact between therapists or other health care practitioners and their clients. J Consult Clin Psychol 52:1054–1061, 1984

Finell JS: Narcissistic problems in analysts. Int J Psychoanal 66:433–445, 1985

Forer B: The taboo against touching in psychotherapy. Psychotherapy: Theory, Research and Practice 6:229–231, 1969

Forer B: The therapeutic relationship: 1968. Paper presented at the annual meeting of the California State Psychological Association, Pasadena, CA, 1980

Freman L, Roy J: Betrayal. New York, Stein and Day, 1976

Freud S: Observations on transference-love (1915), in Complete Psychological Works, standard ed, Vol 12. Translated and edited by Strachey J. London, Hogarth Press, 1958, pp 157–173

Freud S: On narcissism: an introduction (1914), in Complete Psychological Works, standard ed, Vol 14. Translated and edited by Strachey J. London, Hogarth Press, 1957, pp 67–102

Freud S: Civilization and its discontents (1930), in Complete Psychological Works, standard ed, Vol 21. Translated and edited by Strachey J. London, Hogarth Press, 1961, pp 57–145

Gabbard GO: The treatment of the "special" patient in a psychoanalytic hospital. International Review of Psychoanalysis 13(3):333–347, 1986

Gabbard K, Gabbard GO: Psychiatry and the Cinema. Chicago, University of Chicago Press, 1987

Gabbard GO, Menninger RW: The psychology of the physician, in Medical Marriages. Edited by Gabbard GO, Menninger RW. Washington, DC, American Psychiatric Press, 1988, pp 23–38

Gabbard GO, Twemlow SW: With the Eyes of the Mind: An Empirical Analysis of Out-of-Body States. New York, Praeger, 1984

Ganzarain R, Buchele B: Countertransference when incest is the problem. Int J Group Psychother 36:549–566, 1986

Ganzarain R, Buchele B: Fugitives of Incest: A Perspective from Psychoanalysis and Groups. New York, International Universities Press, 1988

Gareffa DN, Neff SA: Management of the client's seductive behavior. Smith College Studies of Social Work 44:110–124, 1975

Gartrell N, Herman J, Olarte S, et al: Psychiatrist-patient sexual contact: results of a national survey. Am J Psychiatry 143:112–131, 1986

Gechtman L, Bouhoutsos JC: Social workers' attitudes and practices regarding erotic and nonerotic physical contact with their clients. Paper presented at the annual conference of the California Society for Clinical Social Work, and the National Federation of Societies for Clinical Social Work, Universal City, CA, October, 1985

Gelinas DJ: The persisting negative effects of incest. Psychiatry 46:312–332, 1983

Geller JD, Cooley RS, Hartley D: Images of the psychotherapist: a theoretical and methodological perspective. Imagination, Cognition and Personality 1:123–146, 1981–82

Gilligan C: In a Different Voice: Psychological Theory and Women's Development. Cambridge, MA, Harvard University Press, 1982

Glaser RD, Thorpe JS: Unethical intimacy: a survey of sexual contact and advances between psychology educators and female graduate students. Am Psychol 41:43–51, 1986

Goedert JJ: Sounding board: what is safe sex? N Engl J Med 316:1339–1342, 1987

Golden JS, Golden MA: You know who and what's her name: the woman's role in sex therapy. J Sex Marital Ther 2:6–16, 1976

Goodchilds J, Zellman G: Sexual signaling and sexual aggression in adolescent relationships, in Pornography and Sexual Aggression. Edited by Malamuth NM, Donnerstein E. Orlando, FL, Academic Press, 1984, pp 233–243

Gottlieb MC, Sell JM, Schoenfeld L: Relationships with patients after termination: clinical, ethical, and legal considerations. Paper presented at the annual convention of the American Psychological Association, Washington, DC, 1986

Greenson R: The Technique and Practice of Psychoanalysis, Vol 1. New York, International Universities Press, 1967

Grubrich-Simitis I: Six letters of Sigmund Freud and Sandor Ferenczi on the interrelationship of psychoanalytic theory and technique. Int Rev Psychoanal 13:259–277, 1986

Hamilton JW: The Doppelgänger effect in the relationship between Joseph Conrad and Bertrand Russell. Int Rev Psychoanal 6:175–181, 1979

Hamilton NG: Positive projective identification. Int J Psychoanal 67:489–496, 1986

Hare-Mustin R: Ethical considerations in the use of sexual contact in psychotherapy. Psychotherapy: Theory, Research and Practice 11:308–310, 1974

Hartlaub GH, Martin GC, Rhine MW: Recontact with the analyst following termination: a survey of 71 cases. J Am Psychoanal Assoc 34:895–910, 1986

Hartman WE, Fithian MA: Treatment of Sexual Dysfunction. Long Beach, CA, Center for Marital and Sexual Studies, 1972

Herman J: Father-Daughter Incest. Cambridge, MA, Harvard University Press, 1981

Herman JL, Gartrell N, Olarte S, et al: Psychiatrist-patient sexual contact: results of a national survey, II: psychiatrists' attitudes. Am J Psychiatry 144:164–169, 1987

Hilberman E, Munson K: Sixty battered women. Victimology 2(3/4): 460–470, 1977–78

Holroyd JC: Erotic contact as an instance of sex-biased therapy, in Bias in Psychotherapy. New York, Praeger, 1983, pp 285–308

Holroyd JC, Bouhoutsos JC: Biased reporting of therapist-patient sexual intimacy. Professional Psychology 16:701–709, 1985

Holroyd JC, Brodsky AM: Psychologists' attitudes and practices regarding erotic and nonerotic physical contact with patients. Am Psychol 32:843–849, 1977

Holroyd JC, Brodsky AM: Does touching patients lead to sexual intercourse? Professional Psychology 11:807–811, 1980

Holtzman BL: Who's the therapist here: dynamics underlying therapist-client sexual relations. Smith College Studies in Social Work 54:204–224, 1984

Horowitz MJ: Stress Response Syndromes. New York, Plenum, 1976

Horowitz MJ: Controls of visual imagery and therapist intervention, in The Power of Human Imagination: New Methods of Psychotherapy. Edited by Singer JL, Pope KS. New York, Plenum, 1978, pp 37–49

Jacobs L, Berscheid E, Walster E: Self-esteem and attraction. J Pers Soc Psychol 17:84–91, 1971

Janis IL: Victims of Groupthink. Boston, Houghton Mifflin, 1972

Jensen SB, Mohl B: Vi er ikke lavet af trae (We are not made of wood), in Parsamtale og Parterapi. Edited by Jensen SB, Hejl B. Copenhagen, Denmark, Munksgaards Forlag, 1987

Jones E: The Life and Work of Sigmund Freud, Vol III. New York, Basic Books, 1957

Kanin EJ, Parcell SR: Sexual aggression: a second look at the offended female. Arch Sex Behav 6:67–76, 1977

Kaplan M: A woman's view of DSM-III. Am Psychol 38:786–792, 1983

Karasu TB: The ethics of psychotherapy. Am J Psychiatry 137:1502–1512, 1980

Kardener SH: Sex and the physician-patient relationship. Am J Psychiatry 131:1134–1136, 1974

Kardener SH, Fuller M, Mensh IN: A survey of physicians' attitudes and practices regarding erotic and nonerotic contact with patients. Am J Psychiatry 130:1077–1081, 1973

Kaufman PA, Harrison E: Open-ended group therapy for victims of therapist sexual misconduct, in Sexual Exploitation of Patients by Health Professionals. Edited by Burgess AW, Hartman CR. New York, Praeger, 1986, pp 173–177

Kernberg OF: Transference and countertransference in the treatment of borderline patients. Journal of the National Association of Private Psychiatric Hospitals 7(2):14–24, 1975

Kernberg OF: Projection and projective identification: developmental and clinical aspects. J Am Psychoanal Assoc 35(4):795–819, 1987

Kilpatrick DM, Veronen LJ, Resnick PA: The aftermath of rape: recent empirical findings. Am J Orthopsychiatry 49:658–669, 1979

Kinsey AC, Pomeroy WB, Martin CE: Sexual Behavior in the Human Male. Philadelphia, WB Saunders, 1948

Kinsey AC, Pomeroy WB, Martin CE, et al: Sexual Behavior in the Human Female. Philadelphia, WB Saunders, 1953

Kohut H: The Analysis of the Self. New York, International Universities Press, 1971

Leiblum SR, Pervin LA: Introduction: the development of sex therapy from a sociocultural perspective, in Principles and Practice of Sex Therapy. Edited by Leiblum SR, Pervin LA. New York, Guilford Press, 1980, pp 1–24

LoPiccolo J: The professionalization of sex therapy: issues and problems, in Handbook of Sex Therapy. Edited by LoPiccolo J, LoPiccolo L. New York, Plenum, 1978, pp 511–526

LoPiccolo J, Heiman JR, Hogan DR, et al: Effectiveness of single therapists vs. co-therapy teams in sex therapy. J Consult Clin Psychol 53:287–294, 1985

Lott AJ, Lott BE: Group cohesiveness, communication level, and conformity. Journal of Abnormal and Social Psychology 62:408–412, 1961

Luepker ET, Retsch-Bogard C: Time-limited treatment groups for patients sexually exploited by psychotherapists, in Sexual Exploitation of Patients by Health Professionals. Edited by Burgess AW, Hartman CR. New York, Praeger, 1986, pp 163–172

Lystad MH: Violence in the Home: Interdisciplinary Perspectives. New York, Brunner/Mazel, 1986

Marmor J: Some psychodynamic aspects of the seduction of patients in psychotherapy. Am J Psychoanal 36(4):319–323, 1976

Masters WH, Johnson VE: Human Sexual Response. New York, Bantam Books, 1966

Masters WH, Johnson VE: Human Sexual Inadequacy. Boston, Little, Brown, 1970

Masters WH, Johnson VE: Principles of the new sex therapy. Am J Psychiatry 133:548–554, 1976

McCartney J: Overt transference. Journal of Sex Research 2:227–237, 1966

Meichenbaum D: Why does using imagery in psychotherapy lead to change?, in The Power of Human Imagination: New Methods of Psychotherapy. Edited by Singer JL, Pope KS. New York, Plenum, 1978, pp 381–394

Miller A: Prisoners of Childhood. New York, Basic Books, 1981

Mills KH, Kilmann PR: Group treatment of sexual dysfunctions: a methodological review of the outcome literature. J Sex Marital Ther 8:259–296, 1982

Moore RA: Ethics in the practice of psychiatry: update on the results of enforcement of the code. Am J Psychiatry 142:1043–1046, 1985

Moteki R: Sexual transference issues for female therapists remain largely unaddressed. Behavior Today, August 1987, pp 2–3

Muehlenhard C, Linton M: Date rape and sexual aggression in dating situations: incidence and risk factors. Journal of Counseling Psychology 34:186–196, 1987

Munich A: Seduction in academe. Psychology Today, February 1978, pp 82–84, 108

Myers MB, Templer DI, Brown R: Coping ability of women who become victims of rape. J Consult Clin Psychol 52:73–78, 1984

Nadelson C, Notman M, Zackson H, et al: A follow-up study of rape victims. Am J Psychiatry 139:1266–1270, 1982

National Association of Social Workers: Code of Ethics of the National Association of Social Workers. Washington, DC, National Association of Social Workers, 1980

National Association of Social Workers: Annual report to the trust: current employment setting, in NASW Data Bank Report 1. NASW Membership–National Summary Tables. Washington, DC, National Association of Social Workers, 1985, p 5

Norman H, Blacker K, Oremland J, et al: The fate of the transference neurosis after termination of a satisfactory analysis. J Am Psychoanal Assoc 24:471–498, 1976

Ogden TH: On projective identification. Int J Psychoanal 60:357–373, 1979

Oremland J, Blacker K, Norman H: Incompleteness in "successful" psychoanalyses: a follow-up study. J Am Psychoanal Assoc 23:819–844, 1975

Perr IN: Statutory rape of an insane person. Journal of Forensic Medicine 13:433–441, 1968

Perry J: Physicians' erotic and nonerotic physical involvement with patients. Am J Psychiatry 133:838–840, 1976

Person ES: Women in therapy: therapist gender as a variable. Int Rev Psychoanal 10:193–204, 1983

Pfeffer A: The meaning of the analyst after analysis. J Am Psychoanal Assoc 11:229–244, 1963

Plasil E: Therapist. New York, St. Martin's/Marek, 1985

Plato: The symposium, in Great Dialogues of Plato. Edited by Warmington EH, Rouse PG. Translated by Rouse WHD. New York, New American Library, 1967

Pope KS: Diagnosis and treatment of therapist-patient sex syndrome. Paper presented at the annual meeting of the American Psychological Association, Los Angeles, August, 1985

Pope KS: Research and laws regarding therapist-patient sexual involvement: implications for therapists. Am J Psychother 40:564–571, 1986a

Pope KS: Therapist-patient sex syndrome: research findings. Paper presented at the annual meeting of the American Psychiatric Association, Washington, DC, May 1986b

Pope KS: Preventing therapist-patient sexual intimacy: therapy for a therapist at risk. Professional Psychology: Research and Practice 18: 624–628, 1987

Pope KS, Bouhoutsos J: Sexual Intimacy Between Therapists and Patients. New York, Praeger, 1986

Pope KS, Levenson H, Schover LR: Sexual intimacy in psychology training: results and implications of a national survey. Am Psychol 34:682–689, 1979

Pope KS, Schover LR, Levenson H: Sexual behavior between clinical supervisors and trainees: implications for professional standards. Professional Psychology: Research and Practice 11:157–162, 1980

Pope KS, Keith-Spiegel P, Tabachnick BG: Sexual attraction to clients: the human therapist and the (sometimes) inhuman training system. Am Psychol 41:147–158, 1986

Pope KS, Tabachnick BG, Keith-Spiegel P: Ethics of practice: the beliefs and behaviors of psychologists as therapists. Am Psychol 42:993–1006, 1987

Pope KS, Tabachnick BG, Keith-Spiegel P: Good and poor practices in psychotherapy: national survey of beliefs of psychologists. Professional Psychology: Research and Practice 19: 547–552, 1988

Rassieur C: The Problem Clergymen Don't Talk About. Philadelphia, Westminster Press, 1976

Raven B, French J: Legitimate power, coercive power and observability in social influence. Sociometry 21:83–97, 1958

Recent ethics cases. Psychiatric News 17(8):8–9, 38, April 1982

Redlich FC: The ethics of sex therapy, in Ethical Issues in Sex Therapy and Research. Edited by Masters WH, Johnson VE, Kolodny RD. Boston, Little, Brown, 1977, pp 232–233

Rhodes ML: Gilligan's theory of moral development as applied to social work. Social Work 30(2):101–105, 1985

Rieker PP, Carmen E: Teaching value clarification: the example of gender and psychotherapy. Am J Psychiatry 140:410–415, 1983

Rinsley D: A contribution to the theory of ego and self. Psychiatr Q 36:96–118, 1962

Robinson WL, Reid PT: Sexual intimacies in psychology revisited. Professional Psychology: Research and Practice 16:512–520, 1985

Rogers C: Client-Centered Therapy. New York, Houghton Mifflin, 1951

Rogers C: A theory of therapy, personality, and international relationships, as developed in the client-centered framework, in Psychology: A Study of a Science, Vol III: Formulations of the Person and the Social Context. Edited by Koch S. New York, McGraw-Hill, 1959, pp 184–256

Rosenfeld A: Incidence of a history of incest among 18 female psychiatric patients. Am J Psychiatry 136:791–795, 1979

Rozsnafszky J: Beyond schools of psychotherapy: integrity and maturity in therapy supervision. Psychotherapy: Theory, Research, and Practice 16:190–198, 1979

Rubin A, Johnson PJ: Direct practice interests of entering MSW students. Journal of Education for Social Work 20(2):5–16, 1984

Santrock JW: Life-Span Development. Dubuque, IA, William C Brown, 1983

Saul LJ: The erotic transference. Psychoanal Q 31:54–61, 1962

Schoener GR: Assessment and development of rehabilitation plans for the counselor or psychotherapist who has sexually exploited clients. Paper presented at the Sixth National Conference of the National Clearinghouse on Licensure, Enforcement, and Regulation, Denver, September 1986

Schoener G, Milgrom J, Gonsiorek J: Responding therapeutically to clients who have been sexually involved with their psychotherapists. Monograph, Walk-In Counseling Center, Minneapolis, 1981

Schover LR: Male and female therapists' responses to male and female client sexual material: an analogue study. Arch Sex Behav 10:477–492, 1981

Schover LR, Jensen SB: Sexuality and Chronic Illness: A Comprehensive Approach. New York, Guilford Press, 1988

Schultz LG: A survey of social workers' attitudes and use of body and sex psychotherapies. Clinical Social Work Journal 3:90–99, 1975

Searles HF: Oedipal love in the countertransference. Int J Psychoanal 40:180–190, 1959

Searles HF: Countertransference and Related Subjects. New York, International Universities Press, 1979

Sechehaye MA: Symbolic Realization: A New Method of Psychotherapy Applied to a Case of Schizophrenia. New York, International Universities Press, 1951

Sell JM, Gottlieb MC, Schoenfeld L: Ethical considerations of social/romantic relationships with present and former clients. Professional Psychology: Research and Practice 17:504–508, 1986

"Sexploitation" by therapists condemned. NASW News, May 1985, p 15

Shepard M: The Love Treatment: Sexual Intimacy Between Patients and Psychotherapists. New York, Wyden, 1971

Shor J, Sanville J: Erotic provocations and dalliances in psychotherapeutic practice. Clinical Social Work Journal 2:83–95, 1974

Siassi I, Thomas M: Physicians and the new sexual freedom. Am J Psychiatry 130:1256–1257, 1973

Simon R: The psychiatrist as a fiduciary: avoiding the double agent role. Psychiatric Annals 17:622–626, 1987

Singer JL, Pope KS: The use of imagery and fantasy techniques in psychotherapy, in The Power of Human Imagination: New Methods of Psychotherapy. Edited by Singer JL, Pope KS. New York, Plenum, 1978, pp 3–34

Siporin M: Moral philosophy in social work today. Social Service Review 56: 516–535, 1982

Smith JT: Medical Malpractice: Psychiatric Care. Colorado Springs, CO, Shepard's/McGraw-Hill, 1986

Smith JT: Therapist-patient sex: exploitation of the therapeutic process. Psychiatric Annals 18:59–63, 1988

Smith JT, Bisbing SB: Sexual Exploitation by Professionals. Potomac, MD, Legal Medicine Press, 1986

Sonne J, Meyer CB, Borys D, et al: Clients' reactions to sexual intimacy in therapy. Am J Orthopsychiatry 55:183–189, 1985

Spencer J: Father-daughter incest. Child Welfare 57:581–590, 1978

Stanton A, Schwartz M: The Mental Hospital. New York, Basic Books, 1954

State punishes therapist sex. NASW News, July 1984

Stoller RJ: Observing the Erotic Imagination. New Haven, Yale University Press, 1985

Stone AA: The legal implications of sexual activity between psychiatrist and patient. Am J Psychiatry 133:1138–1141, 1976

Stone LG: A study of the relationships among anxious attachment, ego functioning, and female patients' vulnerability to sexual involvement with their male psychotherapists. Unpublished doctoral dissertation, California School of Professional Psychology, Los Angeles, 1980

Stone MH: Management of unethical behavior in a psychiatric hospital staff. Am J Psychother 29:391–401, 1975

Sullivan HS: The Psychiatric Interview. New York, WW Norton, 1954

Taylor B, Wagner N: Sex between therapists and clients: a review and analysis. Professional Psychology 7:593–601, 1976

Tennov D: Love and Limerence: The Experience of Being in Love. New York, Stein and Day, 1979

Vaillant G, Sobowale N, McArthur C: Some psychologic vulnerabilities of physicians. N Engl J Med 287:372–375, 1972

Verhulst J: Limerence: notes on the nature and function of passionate love. Psychoanalysis and Contemporary Thought 7(1):115–138, 1984

Vinson JS: Sexual contact with psychotherapists: a study of client reactions and complaint procedures. Unpublished doctoral dissertation, California School of Professional Psychology, Los Angeles, 1984

Voth H: Love affair between doctor and patient. Am J Psychother 26:394–400, 1972

Walker E, Young PD: A Killing Cure. New York, Holt, Rinehart, & Winston, 1986

Walster E: The effect of self-esteem on romantic liking. J Experimental Soc Psychology 1:184–197, 1965

Webb W: The doctor-patient covenant and the threat of exploitation. Am J Psychiatry 143:1149–1150, 1986

Weiner, MF: Health and pathological love: psychodynamic views, in On Love and Loving: Psychological Perspectives on the Nature and Experience of Romantic Love. Edited by Pope KS. San Francisco, Jossey-Bass, 1980, pp 114–132

Wheelis A: The Doctor of Desire. New York, WW Norton, 1987

Whittington H: Therapy's tender trap—the analyst as fantasy lover. Savvy, June 1981, pp 50–54

Winnicott DW: The Maturational Processes and the Facilitating Environment. New York, International Universities Press, 1965

Zelen S: Sexualization of therapeutic relationships: the dual vulnerability of patient and therapist. Psychotherapy: Theory, Research and Practice 22:178–185, 1985

Zentner EB, Pouyat SB: The erotic factor as a complication in the dual-sex therapy team's effective functioning. J Sex Marital Ther 7:114–121, 1978

Zilbergeld B: Male Sexuality. New York, Bantam Books, 1978

Index